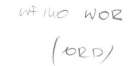
There's a Lot of it About

Acute respiratory infections in primary care

Graham Worrall, MBBS, MSc, MRCGP, FCFP
Professor of Family Medicine, Memorial University of Newfoundland
Director, Centre for Rural Health Studies, Whitbourne, Newfoundland

Forewords by

Chris Del Mar

and

James Hutchinson

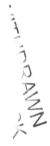

Radcliffe Publishing
Oxford • Seattle

Radcliffe Publishing Ltd
18 Marcham Road
Abingdon
Oxon OX14 1AA
United Kingdom

www.radcliffe-oxford.com
Electronic catalogue and worldwide online ordering facility.

British Library Cataloguing in Publication Data

A catalogue record for this book is available from the British Library.

ISBN-10 1 84619 084 3
ISBN-13 978 1 84619 084 1

Typeset by Anne Joshua & Associates, Oxford
Printed and bound by TJ International Ltd, Padstow, Cornwall

To my dear wife Sylvia, who has endured several years of
my obsessive interest in coughs and colds.

Contents

Forewords   vi
About the author   viii
Acknowledgements   ix

 1 Introduction   1

 2 The epidemiology and aetiology of acute respiratory
   infections seen by GPs in the developed world   7

 3 The common cold   15

 4 Acute sore throat   24

 5 Acute otitis media   37

 6 Acute sinusitis   49

 7 Acute bronchitis   58

 8 Influenza   67

 9 Croup   80

10 Bronchiolitis   90

11 Clinical judgement versus diagnostic tests   102

12 Antibiotic prescribing and resistance   111

13 Strategies for promoting change   123

Index   139

Foreword

It is not often that one can pick up a book designed for doctors about diseases so common we see them every day, and, moreover, every single one of us experiences regularly. Of course, the corollary is that we doctors might think we know all about these acute respiratory diseases. If it is true that familiarity breeds contempt, then we will understand why it is that we give these diseases less intellectual fire-power than they deserve. Underestimating them might be one of the most serious mistakes we could make: witness the increasing anxieties that acute respiratory infections in the form of the recent SARS coronavirus, and 'bird flu' (H5N1 disease) threats.

But this is not the only reason for underestimating the importance of the whole group of diseases: new ways of thinking about the impact of illness on our society in the form of *burden of disease* make us realise that illnesses that affect large numbers of the population can often have as much impact as more deadly but much rarer ones.

There is much more to these diseases than most of us realise. It will not take you long to find fascinating and useful material here. The material is set out to make a story out of the generation of the incomplete knowledge we have. So it makes for a very interesting read.

The evidence about management, as well as diagnosis, is very important. Acute respiratory infection is one of the important areas in which mistaken beliefs about the benefits of antibiotics, not only by our patients, but also by us doctors, probably contribute to the development of bacterial resistance. Graham Worrall has highlighted new forms of treatment that we often forget when we reach for the pad to write another 'safety' prescription for antibiotic.

So, read on: there is a wealth of information here.

Chris Del Mar MD FRACGP MA MB BChir FAFPHM BSc
Dean of Health Sciences and Medicine
Coordinating Editor of the
Cochrane Acute Respiratory Infections Review Group
Bond University, Gold Coast, Australia
August 2006

Foreword

The most important world public health problem – that is what many notable authorities have called antibiotic resistance. And, despite myriad dire warnings, study after study has described 'inappropriate' antibiotic prescribing. Having spent much time considering the reasons for this apparent paradox, my focus naturally became acute respiratory tract infections in primary care, as there certainly is 'a lot of it about'. Ninety percent of antibiotics are prescribed in outpatient settings and three quarters of those prescriptions are for respiratory tract infections. How do we help physicians to become conservative, careful prescribers?

The cornerstone to any lasting behavioral change is education. *There's a Lot of it About – Acute respiratory infections in primary care* is an objective, thoughtful treatment of a subject that accounts for a large part of a primary care physician's working life but inexplicably little of his or her training. Thorough evaluation of the literature, often exposing huge gaps in the study of these extremely common conditions, will serve as an impetus for study and a guide to rational decision-making. The straightforward approach with excellent practical distillations of the evidence and resulting recommendations is perfect for the busy physician or busy student.

As someone who teaches medical students about infections I have longed for a concise resource to support my efforts at encouraging prudent antibiotic prescription for respiratory tract infections. I long no more.

Jim Hutchinson
Associate Professor of Medicine
Microbiology and Infectious Diseases
Department of Microbiology
Health Sciences Center
St. John's, NL, Canada
August 2006

About the author

Graham Worrall received his medical training at the Royal Free Hospital in the United Kingdom and his epidemiology training at McMaster University, Canada. He has been a general practitioner for 30 years, firstly in urban Yorkshire, England and then in Newfoundland, Canada. He is currently a Professor of Family Medicine and the Family Medicine Research Director at Memorial University of Newfoundland, Canada and also the Director of the Centre for Rural Health Studies in Whitbourne, Newfoundland, where he still works as a country doctor.

Acknowledgements

Most of the writing of this book was done during a sabbatical year spent in Australia and the UK. While studying the enormous literature on the common respiratory infections, I received advice and encouragement from many people. I have tried to mention them all below, and apologise for any omissions.

Australia: Jeremy Anderson, Institute of Health Services Research; Sally Green, Australasian Cochrane Centre; staff of Hargrave–Andrew Library, Monash University; Claire Harris, Centre for Clinical Effectiveness, Monash Medical Centre; staff of the Australasian Cochrane Centre, Melbourne; Chris del Mar, Bond University.

United Kingdom: Jos Kleijen, Centre for Reviews and Dissemination, York University; Ian Watt, Centre for Health Sciences, York University; Nicky Britten, Peninsula Medical School; Chris Butler, University of Cardiff Medical School; staff of Centre for Reviews and Dissemination, York University.

Canada: Jim Hutchinson, Infectious Diseases Control, Memorial University of Newfoundland and Labrador, St John's; staff of Health Sciences Center Library, St. John's.

Chapter 1

Introduction

Next to hangovers, women and taxes, these [respiratory tract infections] are man's most important affliction.

Prof. Alfred Evans

Diseases: the more common they are, the less they are studied.

Dr Robert de Melker

- Acute respiratory infections are the most common conditions seen by family doctors and primary healthcare workers.
- They account for one-quarter of adult visits.
- They account for one-third of childhood visits.
- They result in one-quarter of all prescriptions.
- They are the leading cause of antibiotic prescriptions.

Like most young family doctors starting work in the community, I was at first surprised by the number of people who came to see me suffering from acute respiratory tract infections (ARIs). In winter, they represented up to a third of my patients, and even in summer they represented a fifth of all the people who visited me. Most of these people did not have the infectious diseases that I had seen and been taught about when I was a medical student and a house officer. There was little meningitis, pneumonia and hepatitis here – just a steady stream of people of all ages and colours, complaining of 'flu', colds, sore throat, earache, cough, sinuses and sniffles.

I rapidly realised that I needed help to manage these ARIs properly. My colleagues and mentors in general practice appeared unflappable in their ability to cope with them, but as time went by, I noticed that each general practitioner (GP) had a different approach to diagnosing and managing these illnesses. They called the same syndromes by different names, they prescribed different medications, they prescribed the same medicines for different durations, and they gave different advice about comfort measures, the prevention of disease spread, and preventive measures for the future. They rarely seemed to be able to explain their actions in a logical way. It seemed clear to me that most of the GPs I observed (both in teaching practices and in the more run-of-the-mill practices where I did locums) had established a treatment regime based upon their own personal experience and, as the ARIs are almost always self-limiting, most doctors found their own idiosyncratic regime entirely satisfactory for themselves and their patients.

Not only was it difficult to find out and understand why they acted as they did, but it soon became apparent to me that (at that time, during the 1970s) little research had been done on these infections, and very little of what had been published seemed relevant to the primary care physician. It was a paradox – the more common the disease, the less it appeared to have been studied.

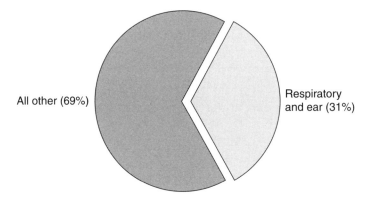

All other (69%)

Respiratory
and ear (31%)

Figure 1.1 Workload of British GPs (Hodgkin, 1978, p. 19).

In my darkness, some beacons shone, including a book entitled *Common Diseases: Their Nature, Incidence and Care*, written by Dr John Fry, a British general practitioner and researcher, who had worked in a suburban practice for over 25 years and built up a unique database of his experience of the common diseases of our communities. He observed that in any two-week period, around one-third of the general population will report experiencing symptoms suggestive of an acute respiratory infection. He also noted that although the majority of people did not consult the doctor about their illness, the minority that did resulted in between a quarter and a third of the general practitioner's workload (Fry, 1974). Seven of the 21 chapters in his book concerned acute respiratory diseases. Soon afterwards, I discovered another seminal primary care research work, *Towards Earlier Diagnosis in General Practice*, by Dr Keith Hodgkin, another British GP who had kept long-term meticulous records of his encounters with all his patients. He gave important advice about the common nature of ARIs in primary care, with hints on how to distinguish self-limiting from serious conditions (*see* Figure 1.1) (Hodgkin, 1978). I was, and remain, profoundly grateful to Drs Fry and Hodgkin.

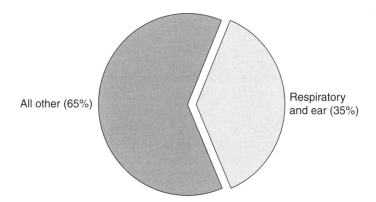

Figure 1.2 Office visits by patient's reason for visit for children under 15 years of age in the USA. From *US National Ambulatory Medical Care Survey, 1995–96.*

I looked further, and discovered that ARIs (including ear infections) accounted for 35% of all office visits for children in the USA (*see* Figure 1.2). Five of the ten commonest diagnoses for children, and three of the top ten for adults in that country, were ARIs. Older textbooks of family medicine, such as *Family Medicine: Principles and Practice* (Taylor, 1988) and *Textbook of Family Medicine* (Rakel, 1984), confirmed the ubiquity of acute ARIs in primary care and devote considerable space to them.

It was striking to me that these traditional textbooks approached the common infectious diseases by stressing that untreated (or inappropriately treated) disease causes significant morbidity, and that the situation could be much improved if family doctors were better at identifying the responsible micro-organism and using the appropriate antibiotic agent. There was little consideration of the epidemiology, mild nature and self-limiting course of most such illness in primary care, and there was little emphasis on the use of watchful waiting and the principle of *primum non nocere* when using powerful pharmacological agents.

More recent texts, such as McWhinney's *A Textbook of Family Medicine* (McWhinney, 1997), quote recent figures from the USA which indicate that sore throats, head colds and cough are the three commonest reasons for visits to primary care doctors (not necessarily all GPs), and from Canada and the UK, where cough, sore throats, colds and earache are all among the top ten most common presenting symptoms.

Since I entered practice, much more research has been done on the diagnosis and management of common conditions, and there is easy internet access to large research databases. There are still many gaps in our knowledge and many areas of controversy, but an increasing knowledge of the principles of research synthesis and evidence-based medicine (EBM) should put primary healthcare workers in a better position than ever to offer their patients with ARIs the best possible care.

Although an article in the *Journal of Family Practice* (de Melker, 1994) bemoaned the fact that 'a scientific basis for the treatment of common diseases is lacking, there are very large gaps in our knowledge, and GP research and training should concentrate much more on these areas', there is now in fact a very large literature on the ARIs.

Aims of this book

> It is easier to buy books than to read them, and easier to read them than to absorb them.
>
> Sir William Osler

First, I look at the epidemiology of ARIs in the developed world and, as a consequence, their impact on the daily work of primary care workers in those countries. This is not as easy as it seems, for two reasons.

1 The ARIs were classified in different ways in different surveys. For example, some surveys included influenza while others did not, some surveys included acute otitis media while others did not, and some studies included 'common colds' while others called them 'non-specific upper respiratory infections.'

2 The healthcare worker of first contact was variously referred to as a 'general practitioner', 'family physician', 'family doctor' or 'primary care physician.' In some systems doctors were working with physician aides, family practice nurses and nurse practitioners.

For the sake of simplicity (and I apologise to all readers who are not doctors), I shall refer to such workers as 'GPs' in this book, except for a few studies (mostly from the USA) where it is clear that the first-contact physician was a paediatrician or an internal medicine specialist. If you work in primary care, this is the book for you.

Secondly, I look at the aetiology of the ARIs in the developed world. This involves more than a simple consideration of which ARI syndromes are likely to be bacterial and which are predominantly viral. It also involves consideration of how GPs can detect the small proportion of ARIs that are bacterial and, indeed, whether it is important for the GP to distinguish between them. I examine whether diagnostic tests for ARIs are available to GPs, and consider their usefulness. I also attempt to examine the natural history of the ARIs, both treated and untreated.

I follow with chapters on the six commonest ARIs in order of decreasing frequency, namely the common cold, acute sore throat, acute otitis media, acute sinusitis, acute bronchitis and influenza. Each chapter is structured in the same way. I look at the epidemiology and aetiology of each specific ARI in more detail, and I discuss the natural history of the illness, usually by looking at the control groups of randomised trials. Then I examine how effective clinical methods and laboratory tests are in helping GPs to diagnose the specific condition. Finally, I look at treatment (both symptomatic and curative) for the condition. Because there are two other ARIs – croup and bronchiolitis – which, although they are not as common, generate high levels of anxiety in both parents and physicians, I have also included chapters on these illnesses.

Because GPs are sometimes criticised for using their clinical judgement alone when diagnosing ARIs, and it has been suggested that more routine testing should be done, I examine what tests are available for the different ARIs. I look at how well clinical judgement compares with the tests, and I consider how feasible and expensive it would be for GPs to use some of the newer technologies and near-patient tests that are now being marketed. I then examine the evidence for the emergence of antibiotic resistance to the bacteria involved in some ARIs, and the effect that antibiotic prescribing by GPs (who prescribe 80% of all antibiotics) may be having on this phenomenon. Although it has been studied most in developed countries, bacterial resistance is a worldwide phenomenon.

Next, I discuss what we know about how GPs treat their patients who present with ARI symptoms. Although there are some differences between doctors in different countries, a surprising uniformity exists. GPs in most countries behave very similarly, and their behaviour has not changed much in the past 30 years. It is well known that GPs prescribe antibiotics more often than the microbial epidemiology dictates. This GP behaviour, which appears irrational at first sight, may be influenced by sensible considerations relating to the method by which the GP is paid, workload factors, diagnostic labelling, doctor–patient relationship factors, GP perceptions, patient expectations, and by the GP judging the potential benefit to the individual patient to be more important than the potential harm to society.

Finally, I consider whether there is evidence that GPs and their patients may benefit from changes in doctor diagnostic and prescribing behaviour. I discuss the literature on attempts to change GP and patient behaviour. If we should change, can we change? Can we persuade our patients to change? And how does the evidence concerning interventions that may cause change relate to the compliance of GPs and patients, and to management guidelines and course of medication?

In each chapter I review the increasing number (sometimes – for example, in sinusitis – almost an excess) of systematic reviews. I did not expect, but soon realised, that several systematic reviews on the same topic, apparently evaluating the same primary research literature, might reach different conclusions. However, as I had expected, many of the better reviews had been undertaken by members of the Cochrane Collaboration. As you probably know, this is an international virtual collaboration of people who seek out and evaluate the best evidence from a massive database of randomised trials of treatment. Not surprisingly, my work quotes heavily from the Cochrane Library of systematic reviews. I also found the US Government's National Guidelines Clearinghouse to be a treasure trove of information about disease management. Visits to either of these sources will richly repay the reader. However, at times I found it necessary to consult the original research papers. I have tried to pay particular attention to those trials that were conducted in primary care, rather than in referral practices or by university-based specialists.

Throughout this exercise, looking at the epidemiology, aetiology and evidence for and against various types of diagnosis and management of ARIs, I have tried to keep in mind the *caritas* which should always inform the *scientia* of general practice. It is well known that high levels of stress and poor levels of social support are related to higher patient use of health services, and greater concern about illness severity. We may be using tests and medicines as placebos in our efforts to help and support our patients, but I think it is important that we realise this is what we are doing, when we do it.

References

De Melker RA, Kuyvenhoven RM (1994) Management of upper respiratory tract infections in Dutch family practice. *Journal of Family Practice*. **38**(4): 353–8.

Fry J (1974) *Common Diseases: their nature, incidence and care*. Medical and Technical Publishing, Lancaster.

Hodgkin K (1978) *Towards Earlier Diagnosis in General Practice*. Churchill Livingstone, Edinburgh.

McWhinney IR (1997) *A Textbook of Family Medicine* (2e). Oxford University Press, New York.

Rakel RE (ed.) (1984) *Textbook of Family Medicine* (3e). WB Saunders, Philadelphia, PA.

Taylor RB (ed.) (1988) *Family Medicine: principles and practice* (3e). Springer-Verlag, New York.

US Center for Health Statistics (2000) National Hospital Ambulatory Care Survey: 2000 Outpatient Department Summary. (www.cdc.gov/nchs/about/major/)

Useful websites

- The Cochrane Library; www.cochrane.org/reviews
- National Guidelines Clearinghouse; www.guideline.gov

The epidemiology and aetiology of acute respiratory infections seen by GPs in the developed world

ARIs are very common in both adults and children. Only a small proportion of people who get these infections choose to attend, or are taken by their parents, to see their GP. Surveys in different countries have found that only 10–15% of sufferers go to the doctor. However, this small proportion makes diagnosing and managing ARIs a large part of the day-to-day work of the GP. This chapter reviews some of the descriptive work on the epidemiology of ARIs, and considers what we know about their aetiology.

Epidemiology

Much of the early epidemiological research on ARIs was done in the UK. Dr Robert Hope-Simpson, a GP in Circencester, formed an Epidemiological Research Unit in his own practice, and for the first time the common ARIs were subjected to systematic study. Hope-Simpson and his team found that 'Colds are endemic, but they and bronchitis are more common in winter. Influenza is epidemic, but is also more common in winter. Tonsillitis and pharyngitis are much less related to seasonal conditions' (Hope-Simpson, 1969).

Pioneering GP researchers studied their own patients (*see* Table 2.1). In England, Dr John Fry found that one-third of the patients on his list would consult him with an ARI each year, and that a GP could expect to see about 15 such people each week (Fry, 1974). Another GP, Dr Keith Hodgkin, found that the seven commonest acute infections seen in general practice were all respiratory (Hodgkin, 1978). Dr Charles Bridges-Webb, an Australian country GP, found that ARIs accounted for about 25% of all episodes of illness that he saw over a 3-year period. Each person had six or seven episodes of ARI per year, and the episodes lasted for 4–10 days. This meant that the average person experienced 50–60 days of respiratory infection per year, and that at any one time 10–20% of the community

Table 2.1 The numbers of people consulting or events occurring in a year in a UK general practice of 2500 patients

Conditions	Patients consulting per year per 2500
Upper respiratory infections	500
Acute tonsillitis	100
Acute otitis media	75
Acute bronchitis and pneumonia	50
Total	725

Source: Fry (1974).

population had an ARI. For adults, the ARIs accounted for 20.8% of all new visits, and for children under 5 years of age they accounted for 46% of new consultations (Bridges-Webb and Dunstone, 1974). Surveys by US and Canadian GPs produced very similar results (Kirkwood *et al.*, 1982; Marsland *et al.*, 1976).

Although only 15% of ARIs cause time off work or school, their frequency means that they are responsible for 50% of all sickness absenteeism. In each year, the average adult takes 5 days off work with ARI, and the average schoolchild takes 11 days off.

The early epidemiological reports by individual GPs have been repeatedly confirmed by larger and more recent studies. A national study of morbidity statistics in UK general practice (McCormick *et al.*, 1995), a study of community-based family practices in the north-west USA (Kirkwood *et al.*, 1982), information from the records of 1000 randomly selected GPs across Australia (Britt and Miller, 2000), and recent data from the Birmingham Research Unit of the Royal College of General Practitioners (which collects information electronically each week from a network of 78 general practices in England and Wales) (Royal College of GPs, 1998) have all confirmed the major role of ARIs in the GP's working day.

Ten most frequent morbidity-related diagnoses for office visits in the USA

Acute respiratory infections, excluding pharyngitis
Essential hypertension
Otitis media and Eustachian tube disorders
Malignant neoplasms
Diabetes mellitus
Chronic sinusitis

Chronic and unspecified bronchitis
Ischemic heart disease
Acute pharyngitis
Non-ischaemic heart disease

Source: US National Centre for Health Statistics (1999).

Ten most frequent morbidity-related diagnoses in children under 15 years of age for office visits in the USA

Otitis media and Eustachian tube disorders
Acute respiratory infections, excluding pharyngitis
Acute pharyngitis
Chronic sinusitis
Chronic and unspecified bronchitis
Asthma
Unspecified viral and chlamydial infections
Streptococcal sore throat
Non-infectious enteritis and colitis
Attention deficit disorder

Source: US National Centre for Health Statistics (1999).

The system in the USA is slightly different to that in most other developed countries, in that a higher proportion of primary care patients is seen by primary care workers other than GPs. Family doctors, paediatricians, nurse practitioners and physician assistants all see the same ARIs, and in the USA about 76 million office visits are made annually for ARIs. The 1999 National Ambulatory Medical Care Survey (US National Centre for Health Statistics, 1999) collected data from office encounters by a multi-stage probability sample of the 18% of US physicians who were in general and family practice. Respiratory and ear symptoms accounted for 17.5% of all office visits (US National Centre for Health Statistics, 1999).

In addition to attending a GP, many people seek care for acute infections in hospital emergency departments. The *US National Hospital Ambulatory Medical Care Survey 2000 Emergency Department Summary* found that respiratory symptoms were responsible for 11.5% of adult ER visits (*see* Figure 2.1) (US National Centre for Health Statistics, 2000). A study in the emergency room (ER) of a children's hospital in Brisbane, Australia surveyed 1000 consecutive patients and found that 40% of those attending had an ARI (Gordon M *et al.*, 1974).

Thus there is strong and consistent evidence that the ARIs are common,

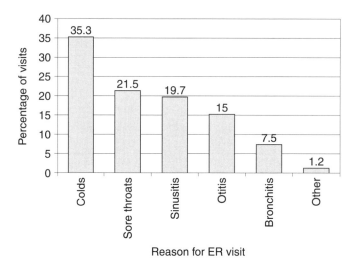

Figure 2.1 Distribution of ARIs attending ERs in the USA. From *2000 National Hospital Ambulatory Medical Care Survey: Emergency Departments.*

and that they account for a large part of the GP workload (*see* Figure 2.2). In developed countries the ARIs represent 15–25% of all first encounters with GPs. The six commonest diagnoses, in descending order of frequency, are colds, sore throat, otitis media, sinusitis, bronchitis and influenza. These are the main conditions that I shall examine in this book. In addition, as mentioned above, I have included chapters on croup and bronchiolitis.

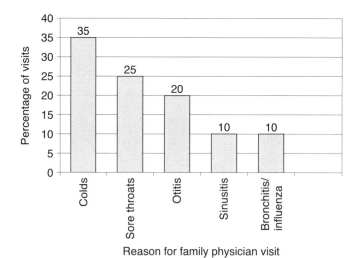

Figure 2.2 Distribution of ARI visits to family physicians: combination of many primary care surveys from the UK, Canada and the USA.

Aetiology

At about the same time that the early epidemiological research on the ARIs was being done, attempts began to determine the aetiology of these illnesses. In 1961–64 in Britain, the Medical Research Council conducted a large study of children under 16 years of age living at home who were suffering from an ARI (Medical Research Council, 1965). Nose and throat swabs were taken from all patients within 4 days of the onset of illness. It was discovered that in only 30% of patients could a virus or a bacterium be isolated, and in 70% of cases no definite organism could be isolated. Even when a virus could be cultured, there was little correlation between the virus and the symptoms. The investigators concluded that 'It is difficult to describe the ARIs very exactly, as there is overlap of symptoms, overlap of signs, micro-organisms are rarely isolated, and the same viruses can produce different syndromes' (Medical Research Council, 1965).

The study of aetiological agents for illnesses in primary care is not easy. Although it may be fairly straightforward to take a swab from the throat or nose, or to obtain sputum, the only reliable way to obtain sinusitis or otitis specimens for culture may be to puncture the tympanic membrane or antral wall. There has been an understandable reluctance to do this, both by academics and by GPs, and the resulting evidence has consequently been scanty. Even when such studies have been done, they are most probably from specialist referral centres with a research interest, and the results are unlikely to represent what happens in primary care. To date, only one ambulatory non-referral study, conducted by Dr Jens Hansen and colleagues in Aalberg, Denmark (Hansen *et al.*, 1995), has used sinus cultures. These investigators persuaded 174 adults with suspected sinusitis to undergo antral puncture. No correlation was found between clinical signs and symptoms, and the results of culture.

The use of cultures to estimate relevant bacterial prevalence in ARIs is also difficult, given the high rates of carriage of potentially pathogenic bacteria. Children in particular appear to have high rates of carriage, approaching 50%. The recovery of pathogenic bacteria from purulent nasopharyngitis specimens and from sputum samples is almost always due to carriage rather than to infection – the isolated organism may not be causing the illness. Similarly, although patients with acute otitis media and acute sinusitis frequently have pathogenic bacteria in the middle ear or sinus cavity aspirates, the majority of these cases (as we shall see) will spontaneously recover without antibiotic treatment, which suggests that in at least a proportion of these cases where bacteria are present, they may not be the agent of infection. Healthy people often carry micro-organisms that have been associated with illness in other people. An Australian study (Bridges-Webb *et al.*, 1971) of the bacteriology of the ENT system took repeated swabs from 138 healthy people and found that it was very common to isolate potential pathogens from the nose, throat and ear, but that there was no relationship between isolation of pathogen and symptoms, and that people with symptoms of ARI were no more likely to yield a positive isolate than people without such symptoms. In total, 50% of healthy people carried potential pathogens in their nose, 30% carried them in their throat and 25% carried them in the external meatus of the ear. There was no relationship between the isolation of pathogens and the presence of disease. The micro-organism profile of individuals with symptoms of ARI did not differ from that of individuals without symptoms. The researchers concluded that 'The flora of the nose and throat has little to do with the occurrence of non-specific ARIs' (Bridges-Webb *et al.*, 1971).

There has also been some justifiable speculation as to whether the ARIs should be classified into discrete entities, or whether they are all part of the same type of infection, being manifested in different parts of the respiratory system. After all, are not the middle ear, throat, nose, sinuses and bronchi all interconnected, like a system of caves? It seems as if a group of common organisms, mostly viruses, can be found in different parts of the cave system in different patients, for reasons which we do not understand. Prominent proponents of this view have been Dr William J Hueston and his colleagues in Charleston, South Carolina. They compared diagnoses of 'acute bronchitis' and 'acute sinusitis' with 'URI' (upper respiratory infections), and found that there is considerable overlap in how GPs record these illnesses in their charts, and that the signs and symptoms that are the strongest independent predictors of 'bronchitis' or 'sinusitis' explain only a small proportion of the variation among illnesses: 'We hypothesize that sinusitis, bronchitis and upper respiratory infections are all variations of the same clinical condition (an acute viral infection) and should be conceptualized as a single clinical entity, with primary symptoms related to different anatomical areas, rather than as different clinical conditions' (Heuston *et al.*, 1998).

Despite some improvement in diagnostic testing and treatment, the situation has not changed much since Dr Alfred Evans, Professor of Epidemiology at Yale University, enumerated the following 'Five Realities' in 1967 (Evans, 1967).

1 The same clinical syndrome may be produced by a variety of micro-organisms. For example, bronchitis has been caused by a wide range of viruses and several different strains of bacterium.
2 The same organism may produce a variety of syndromes. For example, *Streptococcus pneumoniae* has been implicated in both acute otitis media and acute sinusitis.
3 The causative organism may differ according to age, time of year and location. Winter and summer croup may be caused by different viruses.

4 Diagnosis of the micro-organism is rarely possible on the basis of clinical findings alone. Viral and bacterial coughs or sore throats are indistinguishable on the basis of clinical signs.

5 The real cause of a large proportion of common ARIs is still not known. Although organisms may be isolated from sick people, it is difficult to ascertain which organism is causing the illness.

Likely causative agents

Despite these difficulties, a large number of studies have attempted to characterise the ARIs by their putative causative micro-organisms, and the consensus is as follows.

- *Common cold* is almost universally caused by rhino- and picornaviruses. Some authorities claim that bacteria may be involved in 5% of colds.
- *Acute sore throat* is usually caused by viruses. Bacteria (mainly Group A beta-haemolytic streptococci) account for 30–40% of cases in children over 5 years of age, and 5–10% of cases in adults and in children under 5 years.
- *Acute otitis media* may be caused by bacteria in up to 65% of cases. Common pathogens include *Streptococcus pneumoniae, Haemophilus influenzae* and *Moraxella catarrhalis*.
- *Acute bronchitis* is predominantly caused by viruses, although 10% of cases may be bacterial. Associated bacteria include *Mycoplasma pneumoniae, Streptococcus pneumoniae, Haemophilus influenzae* and *Moraxella catarrhalis. Chlamydia pneumoniae* and *Bordetella pertussis* may occur.
- *Acute sinusitis* may be caused by bacteria in up to 40% of cases. Common pathogens include *Streptococcus pneumoniae, Haemophilus influenzae* and *Moraxella catarrhalis*.
- *Influenza* is usually caused by influenza A and B viruses.
- *Croup* is most commonly caused by parainfluenza viruses 1 and 3, although influenza A and B viruses, adenovirus and respiratory syncytial virus can cause some cases.
- *Bronchiolitis* is usually caused by respiratory syncytial virus.

Despite the doubts that some authors have about the nosology of the ARIs, I have decided to discuss them by the usual diagnostic categories. As each ARI is discussed, its overlap with the other ARIs, its diagnosis and its likely aetiology will be covered.

References

Bridges-Webb C and Dunstone MW (1974) The Australian General Practice Morbidity and Prescribing Survey 1969–74. Aspects of morbidity: respiratory infections. *Med J Aust.* **2 (Suppl. 1)**: 18–20.

Bridges-Webb C, Gulasekharam J and Graydon JJ (1971) A bacteriological study of the upper respiratory tract of healthy people. *Med J Aust.* **1**: 735–8.

Britt HC and Miller GC (2000) The BEACH study of general practice. *Med J Aust.* **173**: 63–4.

Communicable Diseases/Morbidity Annual Report. Royal College of General Practitioners, Birmingham Research Unit (1998). PHLS, London.

Evans AS (1967) Clinical syndromes in adults caused by respiratory illness. *Med Clin N America.* **51**: 803–18.

Fry J (1972) Twenty-one years in general practice – changing patterns. *J R Coll Gen Pract.* **22**: 521–8.

Fry J (1974) *Common Diseases: their nature, incidence and care.* MTP Medical and Technical Publishing, Lancaster.

Gordon M, Lovell S and Dugdale AE (1974) The value of antibiotics in minor respiratory illness in children: A controlled trial. *Med J Aust.* **1**: 304–6.

Hanson JG, Schmidt H, Rosberg J *et al.* (1995) Predicting acute maxillary sinusitis in a general practice population. *BMJ.* **311**: 233–6.

Hodgkin K (1978) *Towards Earlier Diagnosis in General Practice.* Churchill Livingstone, Edinburgh.

Hope-Simpson RE (1969) A respiratory virus study in Great Britain: review and evaluation. *Prog Med Virol.* **11**: 354–407.

Hueston WJ, Eberlein C, Johnson, D and Mainous AG (1998) Criteria used by clinicians to differentiate sinusitis from viral upper respiratory tract infection. *J Fam Pract.* **46**: 487–92.

Kirkwood CR, Clure HR, Brodsky R *et al.* (1982) The diagnostic content of family practice: 50 most common diagnoses recorded in the WAMI community practices. *J Fam Pract.* **15**: 485–92.

McCormick A, Fleming D and Charlton J (1995) *Morbidity Statistics from General Practice, Fourth National Survey 1991–92.* HMSO/Office for National Statistics, London.

Marsland DW, Wood M and Mayo F (1976) Content of family practice. Part 1. Rank order of diagnoses by frequency. *J Fam Pract.* **3**: 37–68.

Medical Research Council Working Group on Acute Virus Infection (1965) A collaborative study of the aetiology of acute respiratory illness in Britain 1961–1964. *BMJ.* **2**: 319–26.

US National Centre for Health Statistics (1999) *Data from the National Ambulatory Medical Care Survey.* www.cdc.gov/nchs/about/major/ahcd/ercharts.htm

US National Centre for Health Statistics (2000) *National Hospital Ambulatory Medical Care Survey: 2000 Outpatient Department Summary.* www.cdc.gov.nchs/about/major/

Chapter 3

The common cold

The only way to treat the common cold is with contempt.
Sir William Osler

Epidemiology and aetiology

- Adults get four to six colds per year, while children get six to eight of them.
- Although most people do not see the doctor when they have a cold, the workload generated by those who do is considerable.
- Colds are the cause of 40% of all time off work.
- Colds are the cause of 30% of all time off school.
- Colds can be caused by over 200 different types of virus, but rhinovirus and coronavirus predominate.

This is the commonest condition that any GP has to deal with. On average, adults get four to six colds per year, while children get six to eight of them. Although most people do not visit their GP every time they get a cold, the small proportion who do generate a lot of work for doctors. Dr John Fry found an incidence of about 500 visits/1000 patients/year (Fry, 1974), which means that a GP may see 10 patients with colds per week, or two per day. Studies have shown that people who visit their doctor with a cold are less likely to have taken an over-the-counter medication (despite all the TV adverts for these products), are more likely to have been sick for 3 or more days, to live in a large household, to be older, to be unhappy or to need a sick note.

The impact of colds on health is substantial. Because colds occur all year round, the burden of illness that they cause is greater than the burden caused by seasonal influenza viruses. Colds account for 40% of all time lost from jobs and 30% of all absenteeism from school.

Much of the early work on the aetiology of the common cold was done in the UK by Dr David Tyrell and his colleagues at the Medical Research Council's Common Cold Unit (CCU) near Salisbury. A former infectious diseases hospital that had many separate and isolated buildings was used to house and, when necessary, to isolate volunteers. Causative viruses were isolated, and volunteers were exposed to viruses, developed colds, and various preventive and curative agents were tried. Over the years, the CCU carried out randomised experiments on 19 911 men and women volunteers. In the USA, much of the early work on the common cold was done at the University of Virginia School of Medicine by Dr Jack Gwaltney and his colleagues. They studied the epidemiology of the common cold and showed that transmission by hand, rather than by droplet, was the most important route of spread. In Australia, a research group led by Dr Bob Douglas at the University of Adelaide conducted a number of treatment and prophylaxis studies of the common cold, using interferon, over-the-counter medications and oral zinc acetate.

There are around 200 viruses that are known to cause colds. Rhino-viruses predominate when the symptoms are mild, and coronaviruses seem to be associated with more severe colds.

When the symptoms are severe, and particularly when they are accompanied by muscle ache and fatigue, influenza and parainfluenza infections should be suspected.

Clinical course and diagnosis

The diagnosis is always clinical.

Only a tiny proportion of cases do not resolve spontaneously.

Complications very rarely occur – usually in infants, the very old, the immunocompromised and chronically ill people.

Symptoms/signs:

- rhinorrhoea
- nasal obstruction
- throat irritation/laryngitis
- cough but normal chest examination
- fever.

Colds last for 5–14 days.

The common cold is a short, usually mild illness in which respiratory and nasal symptoms, such as runny nose, are the most frequent. Other symptoms, such as malaise, may also be present. Symptoms caused by colds typically last for 1–2 weeks, and most patients will feel better after the first week. Most cases resolve spontaneously, although a very small proportion become complicated by bacterial sinusitis, otitis or pneumonia. This is most likely to occur in infants, the elderly and people who are immunocompromised or chronically ill, but there is no reliable way to predict who will fare poorly (National Guidelines Clearinghouse, 2001; Tyrell and Fry, 1975).

Tests are of no use in diagnosing the common cold. The diagnosis is usually certain when the patient presents with an acute illness with symptoms and signs referable predominantly to the nasal passage, sometimes with a cough, with or without fever. The infection is a self-limiting illness, typically lasting for 5–14 days (with a peak at 3–5 days). The onset of symptoms is rapid. Nasal discharge is initially clear and often becomes yellow or green towards the end of the infection. The presence of yellow or green discharge is not an indication of bacterial infection. It occurs when leucocytes are destroyed while fighting the infection.

Treatment

- Antitussives relieve cough in adults.
- Over-the-counter cough syrups relieve symptoms in schoolchildren.
- There is no evidence for the efficacy of over-the-counter medication in preschool children.
- There is no evidence of benefit from treatment with antihistamines.
- Decongestants relieve cold symptoms.
- Antipyretics/non-steroidal anti-inflammatory drugs (NSAIDs) may relieve fever and headache, but do not affect the clinical course.
- *Echinacea*: no evidence of effect in treating colds.
- *Vitamin C*: may reduce duration by less than half a day.
- *Zinc*: may reduce the duration of a cold slightly, but there is no consistent evidence of benefit.
- *Comfort measures*: steam inhalation relieves symptoms, but there is no good evidence for other comfort measures.
- *Antibiotics*: no evidence of effectiveness.

It cannot be overemphasised that there is no effective treatment for the cold, despite many claims.

We shall now look at the various preparations that people take, often in an attempt to relieve the symptoms rather than cure the illness.

Antitussives

It has been estimated that 75% of us take an antitussive when we get a cold. Nevertheless, despite their ubiquitous presence in the drug stores and their almost universal use, there is not much evidence that antitussives actually work. Trials of the ingredient agents, such as dextromorphan, codeine and ipratropium, have not been convincing, nor is there evidence that the expectorants, such as guaifenesin, help the patient to get better more quickly. Antitussives are more effective in adults than in children, and codeine is likely to have unpleasant side-effects in young children. Several extensive reviews of these agents have concluded that the best that can be said for them is that they ease the symptoms of some people until the cold gets better (ICSI, 2001; Schroeder and Fahey, 2002).

Antihistamines

These have been the subject of a number of well-designed studies, but reviewers have concluded that the literature offers little support for the use of antihistamines in the common cold. One well-conducted systematic review by Dr Paul Luks of the Montefiore Medical Center, New York, found that compared with placebo, antihistamines reduced symptoms of runny nose and sneezing for the first 2 days of both naturally occurring and experimentally induced colds (Luks and Anderson, 1996).

Decongestant

A Cochrane Review of over-the-counter medications by Dr Knut Schroeder at the University of Dundee (Schroeder and Fahey, 2002) found that a single dose of nasal decongestant reduced subjective symptom scores by 13%, but there was no evidence of benefit from repeated use over several days. Nasal sprays or decongestants may provide temporary relief of symptoms. Another Cochrane Review of nasal decongestants for the common cold in adults, by Dr David Taverner at the University of Adelaide (Taverner *et al.*, 1999), found that there was a 13% reduction in symptom score after administration of decongestants, compared with placebo. There was a significant initial decrease in airways nasal resistance when agents such as oxymetazoline, norepinephrine and pseudoephedrine were used. However, there was no significant decrease in congestion after repeated doses of decongestant over a 5-day period. It is well known that long-term use of nasal decongestants can lead to the development of rhinitis medicamentosa.

Antipyretics/NSAIDs

These have been found to relieve the headaches and sore throats associated with a cold, but they do not shorten the duration of the illness.

Echinacea

Extracts from the *Echinacea* plant are widely used by patients and practitioners in Europe and the USA, both to prevent and to treat upper respiratory tract infections. In Germany alone there are currently more than 200 preparations on the market that contain extracts of Echinacea, either alone or in combination with other plant products. A systematic review by Dr Dieter Melchart and colleagues at the University of Munich found that most trials reported favourable results and, overall, the results suggested that some Echinacea preparations may be more effective than placebo. However, the reviewers concluded that as yet there is insufficient evidence to recommend a specific Echinacea preparation, as the products varied widely in strength and formulation (Melchart *et al., 2002)*.

Vitamin C

Vitamin C has also been popular in the prevention and treatment of colds, especially since the publication of books by Dr Linus Pauling (Pauling, 1971). There have been two systematic reviews of the vitamin C trials (Douglas *et al.,* 1997; Hermila, 1996). They found that there was a consistently modest therapeutic effect, with shortening of the duration of symptoms by about half a day. Some small studies have explored the effect of vitamin C when people are under extreme physical stress (e.g. during military training or long-distance running). The vitamin may have a small preventive effect in individuals who are predisposed to recurrent colds.

Zinc

It is known that zinc possesses some antiviral properties *in vitro*, so the treatment has biological plausibility. Since the publication of the results of a randomised controlled trial of zinc lozenges conducted in 1983 by Dr George Eby and colleagues (Eby *et al.,* 1984) which suggested that the treatment could cut the duration of cold symptoms by almost half, there has been much interest in the use of zinc lozenges for the common cold. Unfortunately, the results of subsequent trials have not been so spectacular. Two reviews of all the zinc trials have been undertaken (Marshall *et al.,* 2001; Garland and Hagmeyer, 1998), and both concluded that evidence for the effectiveness of zinc lozenges in reducing the duration of common colds is lacking. They comment that even if the use of zinc produces a modest reduction in severity and duration of symptoms, it must be weighed against the unpleasant taste of zinc and the need to administer it frequently.

Antiviral agents

There have been many studies of antiviral medications, such as interferon and interferon inducers, for the common cold. Unfortunately, according to a heroic review by Jefferson and Tyrell (2001), who examined 241 studies, any slight beneficial effect that such agents have on colds is outweighed by their unpleasant side-effects.

Comfort measures

Mothers around the world have traditionally recommended comfort measures for colds. Humidification of the environment, plentiful warm fluids, a nutritious diet, throat lozenges, salt-water gargles, saline nose drops, elevation of the head of the bed and adequate rest have all been advocated. Steam inhalation does serve as an effective comfort measure for some people. There have been several trials of steam inhalation. A systematic review of six trials supported the use of warm vapour inhalations to relieve symptoms of the common cold (Singh, 2001).

Antibiotics

It seems clear that, despite claims for vitamin C, echinacea and zinc, there is little evidence that they represent effective treatments for the common cold. Perhaps this is why repeated studies have shown that physicians persist in prescribing antibiotics – a triumph of hope over experience – for people with colds. Reports from the USA, the UK, Australia, New Zealand, the Netherlands, Finland, Italy, Croatia and Taiwan have all shown that GPs prescribe antibiotics for up to half of all patients they see with the common cold. In other countries, patients are able to buy antibiotics for themselves. Although three-quarters of the world's population live in Africa, the Middle East, South America and Asia, these countries together account for only about 20% of the world's antibiotic consumption. Physicians in the developed world are responsible for the bulk of antibiotic prescribing.

A Cochrane Review of antibiotics and the common cold, undertaken by New Zealand GP Bruce Arroll, concluded that antibiotics have no effect on the severity or duration of the cold (Arroll and Kenealy, 2002). Most of the nine trials in the review were not conducted in general practice – they used ER patients, young military recruits or people attending infectious diseases clinics. Of the two trials that were conducted in general practice, neither Dr John Howie's study of men in Glasgow (Howie and Clark, 1970) nor Dr John Taylor's study of children aged 2–10 years in general practice in the UK (Taylor *et al.*, 1977) showed any benefits from the use of antibiotics.

Ever since the pronouncement by the seventeenth-century Sage of Leyden, Gerardus van Swieten, '*Certum est, quod in omnibum pectoris morbis, sputa attentam moreatur considerationem*' (It is certain that, in considering all chest diseases, careful attention must be paid to the sputum), doctors have been paying far too much attention to sputum and snot. Many patients, and regrettably also many doctors, still think that green or purulent sputum or nasal discharge is a justification for the use of antibiotics. However, this sign does not mean that a cold needs antibiotics, as it does not discriminate between viral and bacterial infection. Purulence occurs when inflammatory cells or sloughed mucosal cells are present, and can result from either type of infection.

Can colds be prevented?

- Hand washing is effective in preventing the spread of colds.
- Echinacea has a possible small preventive effect.
- Vitamin C has no effect.
- Ginseng may have a small effect.
- There are no effective vaccines.

As it seems clear that colds cannot be cured, much effort has been expended in trying to prevent them. Several studies (none of them well-designed trials) have found that hand washing is the most effective way to prevent the spread of the common cold, especially at the onset of the illness or when the patient is febrile, when the cold is most contagious.

Echinacea

A review of the many studies of preventive effects of regular administration of Echinacea concluded that, despite the generally poor quality of the trials, slightly fewer people had colds when they took the preparation (Melchart, 2002).

Vitamin C

Two reviews of the effects of taking preventive vitamin C found that there was no beneficial effect for most people, although there may be small subgroups (such as competitive athletes and those doing heavy physical work) who might benefit (Douglas *et al.*, 1997; Hermila, 1997)

Ginseng

A recent study conducted in Alberta, Canada, compared people who took two capsules of North American ginseng extract daily for 4 months during the winter season with controls (Predy *et al.*, 2005). Ginseng appeared to reduce the mean number of colds caught, the proportion of individuals who had more than two colds and the duration of the cold symptoms. More research is needed to confirm the findings of this study. Whether many people are prepared to take relatively expensive medicines regularly throughout the cough and cold season each year, in the hope of gaining a modest preventive benefit, remains to be seen.

Vaccines

At present there are no effective vaccines for the common cold. Some of the earliest recorded trials of the prevention of common colds tried using vaccines, but found that they were not effective (Scientific Committee on Common Cold Vaccines, 1965; Ferguson *et al.*, 1927)

References

Arroll B and Kenealy T (2002) Antibiotics for the common cold (Cochrane Review). In: *The Cochrane Library. Review CD000247.* Update Software, Oxford.

Douglas RM, Chalker EB and Treacy B (1997) Vitamin C for preventing and treating the common cold (Cochrane Review). In: *The Cochrane Library. Review CD000980.* Update Software, Oxford.

Eby GA, Davis ER and Halcomb WW (1984) Reduction of duration of common cold by zinc gluconate lozenges in a double-blinded study. *Antimicrob Agents Chemotherapy.* **25**: 20–4.

Ferguson FR, Davy AFC and Topley WW (1927) The value of mixed vaccines in the prevention of the common cold. *J Hygiene.* **26**: 98–109.

Fry J (1974) *Common Diseases: Their nature, incidence and care.* Medical and Technical Publishing, Lancaster.

Garland ML and Hagmeyer KO (1998) Role of zinc lozenges in treatment of the common cold. *Annals of Pharmacotherapy.* **32**: 63–9.

Hermila H (1996) Vitamin C and common cold incidence: a review of studies with subjects under heavy physical stress. *Int J Sports Med.* **17**(5): 379–83.

Howie JG and Clark GA (1970) Double blind trial of dimethyl tetracycline in minor respiratory illness in general practice. *Lancet.* **2**: 99–102.

Institute for Clinical Systems Improvement (2001) *Viral Upper Respiratory Tract Infections in Children and Adults.* ICSI, Bloomington, MN.

Jefferson TO and Tyrell D (2001) Antivirals for the common cold (Cochrane Review). In: *The Cochrane Library. Review CD002743.* Update Software, Oxford.

Luks D and Anderson MR (1996) Antihistamines and the common cold: a review and critique of the literature. *J Gen Intern Med.* 11: 240–44.

Marshall I (2001) Zinc for the common cold (Cochrane Review). In: *The Cochrane Library. Review CD001364.* Update Software, Oxford.

Melchart D, Linde K, Fischer P and Kaesmayr J (2002) Echinacea for the common cold (Cochrane Review). In: *The Cochrane Library. Review CD000530.* Update Software, Oxford.

National Guidelines Clearinghouse (2001) *Viral Upper Respiratory Tract Infections (VURTIs) in Children and Adults.* Institute for Clinical Systems Improvement, Bloomington, MN.

Pauling L (1971) Ascorbic acid and the common cold. *Am J Clin Nutrition.* 24: 1294–9.

Predy GN, Goel V, Lovlin R *et al.* (2005) Efficacy of an extract of North American ginseng containing polyfuranosyl-pryanosyl-saccharides for preventing upper respiratory tract infections: a randomised controlled trial. *Can Med Assoc.* 173: 1043–8.

Schroeder K and Fahey T (2002) Over-the-counter medications for acute cough in children and adults in ambulatory settings (Cochrane Review). In: *The Cochrane Library. Review CD001831.* Update Software, Oxford.

Scientific Committee on Common Cold Vaccines (1965) Prevention of colds by rhinovirus vaccination. *BMJ.* 1: 1344–9.

Singh M (2002) Heated humidified air for the common cold (Cochrane Review). In: *The Cochrane Library. Review CD001728.* Update Software, Oxford.

Taylor B, Abbott GD, Kerr MM and Ferguson DM (1977) Amoxycillin and co-trimoxazole in presumed viral respiratory infections in childhood. *BMJ.* 2: 552–4.

Taverner D, Bickford L and Draper M (1999) Nasal decongestants for the common cold (Cochrane Review). In: *The Cochrane Library. Review CD001953.* Update Software, Oxford.

Tyrell DAJ and Fry J (1975) *Common Colds and Related Diseases.* Edward Arnold, London.

Chapter 4

Acute sore throat

*The pharynx is the garbage dump of the bronchial tubes and the nasal
passages.*

Sir William Osler

Epidemiology and aetiology

- Sore throat is the second commonest acute infection seen by GPs.
- Less than 1 in 10 people with a sore throat go to see their GP.
- Sore throat is predominantly a disease of youth and the early
  school years.
- Sore throats are more common in autumn and winter.

Acute sore throat accounts for 1–2% of all outpatient visits, whether to
GPs' surgeries or to ER departments, and about 4% of all GP visits.
Although family doctors may sometimes be tempted to believe otherwise,
only a small proportion of people with sore throats seek medical attention.
In Canada, only 8% of sore throats lead to a physician visit (McIsaac *et al.*,
1997) and the corresponding figure in the Netherlands is 9% (Dagnelie *et
al.*, 1994). It has been found that people who rated their sore throat as 4 or
5 on a 5-point severity scale were more likely to visit the doctor, but still
only 50% of them sought medical help (McIsaac *et al.*, 1997).

- Viruses are responsible for 85–95% of adult sore throats.
- Viruses cause 70% of sore throats in children aged 5–16 years.
- Viruses cause 95% of sore throats in children under 5 years of age.
- The commonest bacterial cause of sore throat is Group A beta-
  haemolytic streptococcus (GABHS).
- At least 30% of GABHS cultured in primary care are due to
  carriers, who are not sick and are at very low risk of infecting
  other people.

A wide range of infectious agents cause sore throat, but viruses are the commonest cause. The most important bacterial cause of a throat infection is Group A beta-haemolytic streptococcus (GABHS), which is responsible for about one-third of sore throats in children aged 5–16 years. In adults and in children aged under 5 years, only about 10% of sore throats are caused by GABHS. Possible non-infective causes of sore throat include postnasal drip, exposure to irritants, smoking and lack of ambient humidity in the home or workplace (ICSI, 2000).

Some people are chronically colonised with GABHS, and these individuals are called carriers. They are not ill, they are at very low risk, if any, of developing suppurative complications, and they are unlikely to spread GABHS to their close contacts. Therefore carriers require no medical intervention. If GABHS grows repeatedly on throat culture, the patient is likely to be a streptococcal carrier. Such a person will not have a raised anti-streptolysin titre, as does a person with an acute GABHS infection, and there will be no response to antibiotic therapy. There are a few rare situations in which identification and eradication of streptococcal carrier states may be desirable – for example, in a family with a history of rheumatic fever, when there has been an outbreak of GABHS in a closed institution, or when tonsillectomy is being considered. In general, however, there is no need to treat carriers.

Clinical course and diagnosis

The typical GABHS patient is a child aged 5–16 years who presents with fairly acute onset of fever and sore throat. A history of streptococcal exposure in the past week may be obtained. A variety of other symptoms, such as headache, nausea and vomiting, malaise, dysphagia and abdominal pain, may be present. Cough and rhinorrhoea are usually absent. Oedema and erythema of the tonsils and pharynx are usually present, the anterior neck glands may be enlarged and tender, and there may be a non-adherent pharyngeal exudate. The breath may be malodorous, and there may be petechiae on the soft palate.

In otherwise healthy people, a sore throat is usually self-limited and rarely produces significant after-effects. A general practice study of acute tonsillitis in 17 countries conducted by the World Health Organization found that, in the vast majority of cases, acute pharyngitis resolved within one week (Green *et al.*, 2004).

Because repeated studies have shown that it is difficult to distinguish between Group A streptococcal and viral infections on clinical grounds alone, earlier guidelines suggested that the diagnosis should be made by culture of throat swabs. Given that the prevalence of GABHS in sore throats seen by family doctors is 10–20%, most sore throats that are seen

- The controversy over clinical diagnosis versus diagnostic testing continues.
- In the relatively low-prevalence primary care situation, both clinical decision rules and laboratory tests result in a large proportion of incorrect diagnoses.
- The consensus on use of clinical signs in adults is that four signs should be used – lymphadenopathy, exudate, fever and absence of cough/runny nose.

  Number of signs   *Course of action*
  0 or 1   No treatment is needed
  2   Consider diagnostic testing
  3 or 4   Treat with antibiotic

- Rapid streptococcal antigen tests take only a few minutes, and have high specificity.
- North American authorities still advocate the extensive use of tests, but they now suggest that there is no need to use throat culture when the rapid streptococcal antigen test is negative. They advocate performing the test on most patients, and treating only those who are positive.
- Some authors suggest that, because of the higher prevalence in this age group, all children aged 5–16 years should be tested.
- Throat culture does not distinguish between acute infection and the carrier state.
- When tests are freely available to GPs, their antibiotic prescribing behaviour does not change much, and any savings resulting from decreased antibiotic use are offset by increased testing costs.

will give negative cultures. In most general practice settings throat culture is rarely undertaken – both the patient and the doctor want a diagnosis and treatment at the first visit. These attitudes have stimulated many research studies. First, attempts were made to identify a constellation of signs and symptoms which would increase the likelihood of GABHS infection being present. More recently, there have been efforts to develop cheap and quick anti-streptolysin tests, which can be used in the doctor's surgery when the patient is first seen. It was hoped that both doctor and patient would be more certain, and happier, that the correct diagnosis and management had been chosen, if good decision rules or precise tests were used.

Sore throat decision rules

Most of the studies to develop sore throat scoring systems were conducted in North America, following the landmark study by Dr Robert Centor and colleagues (Centor *et al.*, 1981) who studied 286 adult patients with sore throats who presented to the Emergency Department at the University College of Virginia. Doctors in Australia, the UK and Europe have also attempted to develop decision rules. There is a large literature on these studies, and the consensus is that the four most useful features to look for are enlarged submandibular glands, an exudate in the throat, the presence of fever, and the absence of cough and runny nose. Other features that make a diagnosis of GABHS unlikely are conjunctivitis, hoarseness, mouth ulcers, a rash and diarrhoea. The four important features are usually used as follows:

- 0 or 1 feature – GABHS infection unlikely
- 2 features – diagnosis uncertain, further testing may be needed
- 3 or 4 features – GABHS infection likely.

Several studies have shown that patients with three or four of these features (who thus have a 'positive' test) are very likely to have GABHS infection. The sensitivity and specificity of the decision rule are 75–80% in these circumstances, compared with the gold standard of throat swab culture results. The rules can be used to identify both patients who were so likely to have GABHS that a confirmatory throat culture is not needed, and those who are so unlikely to have GABHS that further testing is unlikely to show a positive result. Using the above rules will successfully identify most patients who need treatment for GABHS infection, while dramatically decreasing excess antibiotic use. A study in Canada (McIsaac *et al.*, 2000) found that use of a clinical score alone, without any rapid testing or culture, would have reduced the prescribing of antibiotics to adults with sore throat by 82% and overall antibiotic prescribing by 88%.

Rapid antigen detection tests

Office testing kits which determine whether a throat swab contains anti-streptolysin antigen are now widely available and are becoming much cheaper. Most rapid antigen detection tests (RADTs) have excellent speci-ficity (> 95%), so false-positive results are unusual. This high specificity is touted as an advantage of the RADTs over clinical rules. Performing rapid antigen testing only in those patients who are symptomatically borderline (with two or three clinical features), and withholding antibiotics from those with negative test results, would substantially decrease antimicrobial prescribing, at the cost of potentially under-treating a small group of patients with GABHS. The RADTs are quick to perform, reduce the need for patient callbacks, allow prompt antibiotic initiation and result in high levels of patient satisfaction. Although throat cultures have higher sensitivity than the RADTs, it has been estimated that 30 cultures would be necessary in order to detect one case of GABHS which the antigen test had missed (Poses *et al.*, 1995).

Decision analysis/cost-effectiveness

The problem of whether to use clinical rules, antigen detection tests or throat swab culture, or some combination of these, has continued to challenge academics. Decision analysis and cost-effectiveness studies have been done in an attempt to determine the best strategy. For a hypothetical 14-year-old patient with a fever and throat exudate, but no cough or rhinorrhoea (in other words, a highly likely suspected GABHS infection), consider the following management possibilities:

1 Treat symptomatically.
2 Treat all such patients with oral penicillin.
3 Treat all such patients with intramuscular penicillin.
4 Do an antigen test, and treat with penicillin only if the test is positive.
5 Do a plate culture, and treat those who are positive after 48 hours.
6 Do a plate culture, and treat all patients immediately with penicillin, but stop therapy if the culture is negative.

Decision analysis and cost-effectiveness studies both indicated that option (4) was optimal in providing the most precise determination of GAHS infections.

What academic studies have not really determined is whether knowledge of the decision rules and use of antigen tests will change the way in which GPs behave. One study of physician use of rapid antigen tests found that doctors frequently prescribed antibiotics even when the test results were negative (McIsaac *et al.*, 1998). Another study found that although use of the sore throat score improved physicians' estimates of the likelihood of GABHS infection being present, it did not alter their use of antibiotics (Poses *et al.*, 1995). At the present time, the best that can be said is that use of the sore throat rules, or the antigen tests, will result in a substantial reduction in throat cultures (in settings where these were commonly done before). However, their use does not guarantee reduced antibiotic prescribing.

The search continues for the optimal approach to this common problem.

Current recommendations

As recently as 1999, both the American Academy of Pediatrics (American Academy of Pediatrics, 1991) and the Canadian Pediatric Society (Canadian Pediatric Society, 1993) were recommending that all children with sore throats should have throat cultures done. Although most authorities do not consider that this is now necessary, there are still some concerns that the decision rules developed from adult populations may not apply to all children. The rules may have to be modified for the paediatric population.

The 2002 Guideline from the Infectious Diseases Society of America (Bisno *et al.*, 2003) updates their 1997 guide. A major substantive change is their acceptance of negative results of RADTs for exclusion of acute streptococcal pharyngitis, without the previously mandated confirmation with a negative culture result. For adult patients, a reasonable approach seems to be as follows.

1 Clinically screen all adults with pharyngitis for the presence of fever, tonsillar exudates, tender or swollen neck glands and the absence of cough.
2 Do not test or treat patients who have none or only one of these features, as they are very unlikely to have GABHS.
3 For patients with two or more of these features, the following strategies are appropriate:
   - test patients who have two, three or four features using a RADT, and limit antibiotic therapy to patients with a positive result
   - test patients who have two or three features with a RADT, and limit antibiotic therapy to patients with positive results; treat all patients who have four features
   - do not use any diagnostic tests, and limit antibiotic therapy to patients who have three or four features.

If testing shows that the sore throat is not caused by GABHS, patients should be educated about the ineffectiveness of antibiotic treatment, the use of home remedies to relieve symptoms, and the actions to take if their symptoms worsen. In patients with exudate, swollen glands, fever and constitutional symptoms, but negative GABHS tests, consider and test for infectious mononucleosis.

Antibiotics and sore throats

If you are still uncertain about the value of antibiotics, even for patients with proven or likely GABHS infection, you can look at a very large sore throat literature. Fortunately, there appears to be only one properly conducted systematic review of the use of antibiotics in sore throat, undertaken for the Cochrane Collaboration by Australian GP Dr Chris Del Mar and colleagues (Del Mar *et al.*, 2000). Once they had excluded older and methodologically unsound studies, they found only nine good-quality studies that had been done in the past 20 years (two studies exclusively on children, three on adults only, and the remaining four on people of all ages). These studies looked at the effectiveness of antibiotic therapy for patients with acute sore throat in general practice settings in the UK, Belgium and the Netherlands, and in primary care walk-in centres and paediatricians' offices in the USA. The review found that antibiotics can have a modest effect on sore throat symptoms. Headache, sore throat and fever were all slightly reduced when antibiotics were taken and, not surprisingly, the effect was greater in patients with positive GABHS tests or culture. The greatest symptomatic improvement associated with antibiotic consumption occurred about 3.5 days into the illness. However, about 90% of treated and untreated patients were symptom-free by the end of 1 week. Antibiotics also shortened the duration of symptoms, but by a mean of only 16 hours overall. The reviewers concluded that antibiotics confer relative benefits in the treatment of sore throat, and that these modest benefits must be weighed against the side-effects of treatment, as antibiotics can cause diarrhoea, rashes and occasionally a severe allergic reaction. The findings of this review were confirmed by another review done in the US (Snow *et al.*, 2001).

Effect of antibiotics on the complications of streptococcal sore throat

Treatment of sore throat with antibiotics:

- does protect against acute rheumatic fever (number needed to treat (NNT) *c*.4000), and may be more effective in developing countries
- does protect against subsequent acute otitis media (NNT *c*.29)
- does protect against subsequent acute sinusitis (NNT *c*.50)
- does protect against subsequent quinsy (NNT *c*.27)
- does not protect against acute glomerulonephritis
- does not protect against subsequent meningitis.

Even if antibiotics have only a slight effect on the symptoms of sore throat caused by GABHS, and the duration of the acute illness, are they effective in reducing both acute and chronic complications?

By comparing the rates of complications that occurred in the placebo groups of the antibiotic trials with those that occurred in the treatment groups, it is possible to estimate whether the antibiotics had a protective effect. Antibiotics reduced the incidence of acute otitis media to about 25% of that in the placebo group (Del Mar *et al.*, 2000). At least 29 people (the number needed to treat, NNT) with sore throat would have to be treated in order to prevent one case of otitis media (which itself is usually a self-limiting condition). The incidence of acute sinusitis was reduced by about 50% (NNT *c.*50). The incidence of quinsy was also reduced (NNT *c.*27). Reviewers have concluded that prevention of these complications in sore throat sufferers in modern Western society can only be achieved by treating many individuals with antibiotics who will derive no benefit from them.

Treatment with antibiotics does not seem to prevent the onset of secondary bacterial meningitis. The same rates of positive blood cultures in children with bacterial meningitis were found in those previously treated and in those not treated with pre-admission antimicrobial agents.

The use of penicillin to prevent acute rheumatic fever (ARF) was hailed as a triumph of early antimicrobial therapy. In 1950, Dr Floyd Denny and colleagues (Denny *et al.*, 1950) conducted a trial of penicillin on 1600 US military recruits with sore throats. ARF developed in only two soldiers who received penicillin, but in 17 of those in the control group. The number of patients who had to take penicillin in order to prevent one case of ARF was *c.*63. However, the incidence of ARF in developed countries has fallen 60-fold since the 1960s, and the number of sore throats that would have to be treated in order to prevent one case of acute rheumatic fever is now estimated to be *c.*4000 (Dajani *et al.*, 1988). Furthermore, rheumatic carditis occurs in only one-third of adults with ARF, and most cases of carditis are mild or non-symptomatic. The number needed to treat in order to prevent one serious case of rheumatic heart disease has recently been estimated to be 12 000–15 000. Although acute rheumatic fever is rare in most populations in developed countries (except for their aboriginal populations), it is still common in the developing world where socio-economic conditions are poor. In these societies, an argument can still be made for more lavish use of penicillin to treat acute sore throats.

Much less academic research has been directed towards considering the risk of post-streptococcal glomerulonephritis, which is very rare, even in the absence of antibiotic treatment. Experts believe that glomerulone-phritis cannot be prevented by treating GABHS.

Treatment of sore throats with antibiotics

- In developed countries, GABHS remains very sensitive to penicillin V.
- Using clinical rules and/or laboratory tests, determine which patients are most likely to have GABHS.
- Consider delaying treatment for 2–3 days, to allow time to observe the clinical course and receive laboratory test results.
- Immediate treatment may increase re-infection rates.
- Treat contacts only during institutional epidemics.
- Giving penicillin twice a day may be as effective as giving it three times a day.
- A 5-day course relieves symptoms as well as a 10-day course, but is less effective in eradicating GABHS.
- Amoxycillin once daily may be sufficient when treating children with GABHS.

Despite considerable evidence that antibiotics have limited use in treating acute sore throat infections, they are often prescribed. Figures from developed countries show that GPs prescribe antibiotics for 50–90% of sore throat patients. If you are a primary healthcare worker and reading this book, you are probably prescribing too many antibiotics for sore throats. Possible reasons for this prescribing 'against the evidence' will be considered in Chapter 12.

If you are going to use an antibiotic for a presumed GABHS sore throat, the drug of choice is still penicillin V. GABHS remains exquisitely and uniformly sensitive to penicillin, and less than 1% resistance has been reported. There has been some debate about the relative merits of pre-scribing penicillin at the first visit, or waiting until throat culture results are available. A trial in Jordan (El-Daher *et al.*, 1991) reported that a higher proportion of children who were treated immediately suffered recurrent infections in the following 4 months compared with those who received delayed treatment. It was suggested that delaying antibiotic treatment for 48–72 hours while awaiting the results of throat culture would significantly reduce the number of patients being treated unne-cessarily, and might be associated with decreased re-infection rates. On the other hand, there have been reports that children with more severe symptoms and higher fevers will experience faster relief of symptoms if they are given penicillin early in the illness. The advent of RADTs and decision rules has probably made these discussions irrelevant.

An open randomised trial conducted in the UK by Dr Paul Little and colleagues compared either immediate antibiotic treatment or antibiotics delayed for 3 days if the symptoms got no better, with no antibiotics at all (Little *et al.*, 1997a). They found that people who took antibiotics were no better by day 3, and did not show a greater improvement in median duration of illness, or in days off school or work, although they did have slightly fewer feverish days. Another contentious issue is how long antibiotics should be taken for, and what the dosing schedule should be, for acute GABHS throat infections. When children in the USA were randomly assigned to receive penicillin for either 5 or 10 days, the patients in each of the two groups got better at the same rate (Gerber and Randolph, 1987). In another trial, children received penicillin once, twice or three times daily. Those on the twice and three times daily regimens recovered equally well, whereas the once daily regimen was not quite so effective (Krober *et al.*, 1990). A meta-analysis has been undertaken of all studies that compared once and twice daily antibiotic dosing for children (Lan *et al.*, 2002). This again suggested that penicillin given twice daily works better than that given once daily. In two randomised trials of adults taking penicillin for either 3 or 7 days, symptoms resolved sooner and more completely in those adults who took the 7-day course of treatment (Schwartz *et al.*, 1981; Zwart *et al.*, 2000).

Another interesting consideration is whether the prescribing of antibiotics to people with sore throats increases the likelihood that they will return to see their doctor for subsequent sore throats. Two British trials (Little *et al.*, 1997a; Little *et al.*, 1997b) have found that prescribing antibiotics, which only marginally affects the resolution of symptoms, enhances the belief in antibiotics and the intention to consult in the future. In other words, people who have had antibiotics once are more likely to return for more.

Treatment of contacts

Streptococcal infection often occurs in epidemics, and contagion is a problem in areas of overcrowding or close contact. Although the American Academy of Pediatrics (1991) recommends antibiotics as a means of reducing spread in schools, the impact on disease spread among non-institutionalised adults is not known. However, it is probably not unreasonable to consider whether an adult who is living in close proximity to small children should also be treated.

Tonsillectomy for recurrent infections

A systematic review was undertaken to determine the effect of tonsillectomy in patients with chronic/recurrent acute tonsillitis (Burton *et al.*, 2000). No trials evaluating the effectiveness of tonsillectomy in adults were identified. Two trials in the USA (Paradise *et al.*, 1984; Paradise *et al.*, 1992) showed that children with recurrent tonsillitis experienced slightly fewer infections in the year following surgery, compared with children who did not undergo tonsillectomy. The benefits must be weighed against the complications of surgery (up to 15% of children had post-operative infections, and up to 4% had haemorrhage).

Non-antibiotic management of sore throats

- Consider non-antibiotic therapy as first-line placebo treatment.
- Non-steroidal anti-inflammatory drugs (NSAIDs) relieve symptoms.

Many trials have looked at non-antibiotic management of throat infections, but few of them are of good methodological quality. Most interventions, such as gargling with salt water, sucking lozenges and eating soft foods, are no more effective than placebo. There has been one systematic review of the effect of non-steroidal anti-inflammatory drugs (Thomas *et al.*, 2000), which they found reduce pain but not illness duration.

Given the evidence for the modest effect of antibiotics on the symptoms and duration of throat infections, primary healthcare workers might consider non-antibiotic therapy as the first-line treatment (knowing that they are probably using a placebo), and check patients if necessary a few days later, to make sure that improvement has occurred.

References

American Academy of Pediatrics, Committee on Infectious Diseases (1991) *Report of the Committee on Infectious Diseases* (22e). American Academy of Pediatrics, Committee on Infectious Diseases, Elk Grove Village, IL.

Bisno AL, Gerber MA, Gwaltney JM, Kaplan EL and Schwartz RH (2003) Practice guidelines for the diagnosis and management of Group A streptococcal pharyngitis. *Clin Infect Dis.* **35**: 113–25.

Burton MJ, Towler B, Glasziou P (2000) Tonsillectomy versus non-surgical treatment for chronic/recurrent acute tonsillitis (Cochrane review). In: *The Cochrane Library, 2003 CD 001802.* Update Software, Oxford.

Canadian Pediatric Society, Infectious Diseases Group (1993) Group A streptococcus: a re-emerging pathogen. *Canadian Med Assoc J.* **148**: 1909–11.

Centor RM, Witherspoon JM, Dalton HP, *et al.* (1981) The diagnosis of strep throat in adults in the emergency room. *Med Decision Making.* **1**: 239–46.

Dagnelie CF, Touw-Otten FW, Kuyvenhovven MM, *et al.* (1994) Bacterial flora in patients presenting with sore throats in Dutch general practice. *Fam Practice.* **10**: 371–7.

Dajani AS, Bisno AL, Chung KJ, *et al.* (1988) Prevention of rheumatic fever. A statement for health professionals from the Committee on Rheumatic Fever, Endocarditis and Kawasaki Diseases of the Council on Cardiovascular Disease in the Young. *Circulation.* **78**: 1082–6.

Del Mar CB, Glasziou PP and Spinks AB (2000) Antibiotics for sore throat (Cochrane Review). In: *The Cochrane Library. Review CD000023.* Update Software, Oxford.

Denny FW, Wannamaker LW, Brink K, *et al.* (1950) Prevention of rheumatic fever: treatment of the preceding streptococcal infection. *JAMA.* **143**: 151–3.

El-Dehar NT, Hijazi SS, Raweshdi MM, *et al.* (1991) Immediate versus delayed treatment of group A streptococcal pharyngitis with penicillin V. *Pediatr Inf Dis.* **10**: 126–30.

Gerber MA and Randolph MF (1987) Five versus ten days of penicillin V therapy for streptococcal pharyngitis. *Am J Dis Child.* **141**: 224–7.

Green LA, Fryer GE, Froom P, *et al.* (2004) Opportunities, challenges and lessons of international research in practice-based research networks: the case of an international study of otitis media. *Ann Fam Med.* **2**(5): 429–33.

Institute for Clinical Systems Improvement (2001) *Healthcare Guideline: acute pharyngitis. General implementation.* (www.icsi.org)

Krober MS, Weir MR, Themelis MJ and Van Hamont JE (1990) Optimal dosing schedule for penicillin treatment for streptococcal pharyngitis. *Clin Pediatr.* **29**: 646–8.

Lan AJ, Colford AM and Colford JM Jnr. (2002) The impact of dosing frequency on the efficacy of 10-day penicillin or amoxicillin for streptococcal tonsillopharyngitis: a metanalysis. *Paediatrics.* **105**: E19.

Little P, Williamson I, Warner G *et al.* (1997a) Open randomized trial of prescribing strategies in managing sore throat. *BMJ.* **314**: 722–7.

Little P, Gould C, Williamson I, Warner G, Gantley M and Kinmonth AL (1997b) Re-attendance and complications in a randomised trial of prescribing strategies for sore throat: the medicalising effect of prescribing antibiotics. *BMJ.* **315**: 350–2.

McIsaac WJ, Goel V, Slaughter PM (1997) Re-considering sore throat, Part I: problems with current practice. *Can Fam Physician.* **43**: 485–93.

McIssac WJ, White D, Tannenbaum D, *et al.* (1998) A clinical score to reduce unnecessary antibiotic use in patients with sore throat. *Can Med Assoc.* **158**: 75–83.

McIsaac WJ, Goel V, To T and Low DE (2000) The validity of a sore throat rule in family practice. *Can Med Assoc.* **163**: 811–15.

Paradise JL, Blustone CD, Bachman RZ *et al.* (1983) Efficacy of tonsillectomy for recurrent throat infection in severely affected children. *New Engl J Med.* **310**: 674–83.

Paradise JL, Blustone CD and Rogers KD (1992) Comparative efficacy of tonsillectomy for recurrent sore throat in more versus less severely affected children. *Pediatr Res.* **31**: 126A.

Poses RM, Cebul RD and Wigton RS (1995) You can lead a horse to water – improving physician's knowledge of probabilities may not affect their decisions. *Med Decision Making.* **15**: 65–75.

Schwartz RH, Wientzen RL, Periera F *et al.* (1981) Penicillin V for streptococcal phayyngo-tonsillitis: A randomized trial of three versus seven days treatment. *JAMA.* **246**: 1790–5.

Snow V, Mottur-Pilson C, Cooper R and Hoffman JR (2001) Principles of appropriate antibiotic use for acute pharyngitis in adults. *Ann Intern Med.* **134**: 506–8.

Thomas M, Del Mar C and Glasziou P (2000) How effective are treatments other than antibiotics for acute sore throat? *Br J Gen Pract.* **50**: 817–20.

Zwart S, Sachs AP, Ruijs GJ, *et al.* (2000) Penicillin for acute sore throat: randomized double blind trial of seven days versus three days treatment or placebo in adults. *BMJ.* **320**: 150–4.

Chapter 5

Acute otitis media

Epidemiology and aetiology

> - Acute otitis media is the second commonest reason for children being taken to see their GP.
> - It accounts for 10–15% of all childhood visits to the doctor.
> - It is the commonest reason for prescribing of antimicrobial drugs.
> - Around 60–85% of children have an attack during the first year of life.
> - After 5 years of age, the incidence rate starts to drop rapidly.

Acute otitis media (AOM) is predominantly a disease of children, in whom it is the second commonest condition to be diagnosed (the common cold being the first). Middle ear infection accounts for 12% of visits to ambulatory healthcare sites for children under 15 years of age in the USA. In Boston, a long-term study of a cohort of 2565 children found that 62% of them experienced an episode of AOM by 1 year of age, and 83% by 3 years (Teele *et al.*, 1989). In the UK, around 30% of children under 3 years of age visit their GP with AOM each year. The peak incidence is between 6 and 15 months.

The most important risk factors for AOM are young age and attendance at day-care facilities or nursery. Other factors include white ethnic origin,

> - Acute otitis media is predominantly a bacterial infection.
> - Viruses may account for a third of cases of AOM.
> - A third of bacterial infections are due to *Streptococcus pneumoniae*, a third to *Haemophilus influenzae*, a sixth to *Moraxella catarrhalis* and the rest to a mixture of species.
> - In small infants, other bacteria, such as *Staphylococcus*, *Klebsiella*, *Pseudomonas* and *Enterobacter* are also found.
> - There is a weak correlation between nasopharyngeal and middle ear bacterial infection.

male gender, and a history of enlarged adenoids or tonsils, asthma, previous episodes of AOM, bottle-feeding, use of a dummy, and a family history of otitis media. Parental tobacco smoking and giving the child a bottle in bed have been associated with a slightly higher rate of otitis media (Uhari *et al.*, 1996).

AOM is the most frequently diagnosed bacterial infection in children. It is usually a bacterial rather than a viral infection. This has been established by performing tympanocentesis on children with ear symptoms (such studies were not conducted in a general practice setting!). American and Finnish children attending ENT clinics underwent tympanocentesis, and bacteria were grown from about 75% of specimens (Gooch *et al.*, 1996; Ruuskonen *et al.*, 1989). The main pathogens were *Streptococcus pneumoniae* (37%), *Haemophilus influenzae* (35%) and *Moraxella catarrhalis* (12%). There was a weak correlation between bacteria isolated from nasopharyngeal swabs and those isolated from the middle ear. In infants during the first few weeks of life, the organisms are less predictable, and may include *Staphylococcus aureus*, *Escherischa coli*, *Pseudomonas aeruginosa*, *Klebsiella* and *Enterobacter* species. However, 20–45% of tympanocentesis specimens culture no organism. The major bacterial pathogens that cause AOM have not changed significantly over the past two decades, and are similar in both adults and children.

Clinical course and diagnosis

- Acute otitis media is usually a self-limited condition.
- In 80–90% of children most symptoms resolve within 3 days, and full recovery within 7 days is the rule.
- In antibiotic trials, the failure rate of treatment group subjects is about the same as the proportion of persistent illness in the untreated placebo groups.
- In developed countries, the incidence of suppurative complications such as meningitis and mastoiditis is now extremely low.

The symptoms of otitis media are earache, discharge from the ear, hearing loss, ear popping, ear fullness, dizziness and fever. Irritability, restlessness, wakefulness and poor feeding may also occur. Pulling at the ears – the symptom beloved of mothers – is not associated with AOM. Earache is a significant predictive symptom for AOM, but may also be a symptom of teething, wax in the ear or migraine.

The natural history of untreated AOM is known from the experience of thousands of placebo-group subjects in antibiotic trials. There is strong evidence that the majority of cases of AOM resolve spontaneously. Three systematic reviews (Rosenfeld, 1999; Marcy *et al.*, 2001; Glasziou *et al.*, 2002) have estimated that in around 80% of children the fever and pain resolve within about 2–3 days, and after 7 days the absence of all symptoms and signs except for middle ear effusion can be expected.

Complications of AOM, although potentially serious, and once moderately common, are now rare in developed countries. A meta-analysis of studies involving 5400 children with AOM, undertaken by Dr Richard Rosenfeld at the Children's National Medical Center in Washington, found no suppurative complications (Rosenfeldl, 1999). It is uncertain whether the decreased incidence of serious complications is due to changes in the natural history of the disease, changes in organism virulence or increases in host resistance. In a Dutch study that evaluated AOM treatment with nose drops and analgesic alone (Van Buchem *et al.*, 1985) none of a total of 4860 children developed meningitis, and only two children developed mastoiditis (which in both cases responded to amoxycillin). The average GP can expect to see serious complications of AOM only once or twice in a 30-year career.

- Diagnosis of AOM is difficult. There is no gold standard for GP diagnosis, and no specific laboratory test for AOM.
- The clinical signs with the highest predictive value for AOM are bulging eardrum, clouding of the eardrum, reduced eardrum mobility and hearing loss.
- Pneumatic otoscopy can reliably distinguish AOM from myringitis.
- Tympanometry and acoustic reflectometry have been found to have high sensitivity and specificity in research studies on paediatric ENT patients, but there are no studies of their value in the typical primary care population.
- In contrast to sore throat, there are no clear clinical decision rules for AOM.

GPs have always diagnosed AOM by looking at the tympanic membrane (TM) for signs that reflect middle ear pathology, namely bulging, redness, and opacity or lack of mobility of the tympanic membrane. Although perforation of the TM with purulent drainage obviously indicates otitis media, erythema may be caused by crying. It is difficult to distinguish between AOM (inflammation and pus in the middle ear accompanied by signs and symptoms of ear infection) and myringitis (inflammation of the tympanic membrane alone or in association with otitis externa).

Dr Pekka Karma, an ENT surgeon in Finland, studied 11 000 children with AOM in order to estimate the predictive value of various clinical signs

(Karma *et al.*, 1993). He found high positive predictive values for a bulging TM (89%), cloudy TM (80%) and impaired TM mobility (78%). Although culture of bacteria from myringotomy fluid is the gold standard for AOM diagnosis, studies using this approach have been conducted in children attending academic centres, with a strong clinical indication for myringotomy. It is worth pointing out that the majority of children with milder disease – who represent the bulk of primary care patients – were not included in diagnostic research studies.

Various technologies have been advocated, usually by specialists, to improve AOM diagnosis by GPs.

Pneumatic otoscopy

Acute AOM is rarely found when TM mobility is completely normal on pneumatic otoscopy. Although most textbooks recommend use of a pneumatic otoscope, few GPs use such an instrument, and no studies have been published comparing regular with pneumatic otoscopy in general practice.

Tympanometry

Tympanometry (which measures the acoustic admittance of the eardrum, which is greatly reduced when the air in the middle ear is replaced by fluid) has a reported sensitivity of 85% and specificity of 80% for the diagnosis of AOM.

Acoustic reflectometry

In acoustic reflectometry a spectrum of sound is reflected back from the TM. A fluid-filled ear reflects back an abnormal amount of sound. An analysis of three outpatient studies involving more than 900 patients, performed by the US Agency for Healthcare Research and Quality (Marcy, 2001) found that acoustic reflectometry had a sensitivity of 90% and a specificity of 86% for diagnosing AOM.

An extensive review (AHRQ, 2002) of various diagnostic instruments for AOM, using myringotomy as the reference standard, and using receiver operating curves (ROC) for sensitivity and specificity, found that pneumatic otoscopy was the optimal diagnostic tool.

In summary, although a diagnosis of AOM is suggested by decreased TM mobility and hearing deficits, as yet there is no scientifically derived and validated diagnostic decision rule for the condition, as there is for sore throat caused by GABHS. Although there are several technologies that improve diagnosis, the only one that seems practicable for primary care work is the pneumatic otoscope, which can reliably detect reduced mobility of the TM. Unfortunately, this tool is rarely used by general practitioners.

There have been no studies of this technique in the uncomplicated GP patient population, using myringotomy as a gold standard. Not surprisingly, family doctors have been reluctant to stick needles through the eardrums of sick children.

Treatment

- Because of the high spontaneous cure rate, there is controversy about the need for antibiotic treatment for AOM.
- Use of antibiotics does not prevent subsequent infections.
- Use of antibiotics does not decrease the number of children with long-term hearing loss.
- Use of antibiotics slightly reduces the duration of clinical signs and symptoms.
    - Full clinical cure is improved by 12% (NNT = 8).
    - Pain is reduced by 4.8% (NNT = 21).
    - Contralateral otitis media is reduced by 5.8% (NNT = 17).
- Use of antibiotics produces side-effects (number needed to harm (NNH) = 11).

In Europe, the role of antibiotics in treating AOM has been controversial since the landmark trial conducted by Louk van Buchem and colleagues in 1981 (van Buchem, 1985). In this Dutch study, only 2.7% of children with otitis media who were treated symptomatically rather than with antibiotics became clinically worse after 3–4 days. Almost all of the children with AOM spontaneously improved. These results confirmed suspicions arising from earlier trials of antibiotic therapy, where it was observed that most of the placebo-group patients were asymptomatic on days 2–7.

Thousands of studies of the treatment of AOM can be found in the literature. However, when systematic reviews and meta-analyses have been undertaken, the majority of these trials have been found to be of poor methodological quality. Unfortunately, different reviewers have applied different criteria and come up with very different numbers of studies to review. Earlier reviews included larger numbers of studies than more recent reviews, which have been conducted with more stringent criteria. This makes comparison of the different reviews difficult.

Nonetheless, the consensus has emerged that there is only weak evidence that routine antibiotic treatment improves the course and outcomes of AOM (Alberta Clinical Practice Guidelines Program 2003). If antibiotics are given as soon as possible after the appearance of AOM symptoms, less than 20% of patients (who cannot be identified, except by waiting) will benefit slightly, and the benefits will only be short-term ones. The most recent and probably the most intensive review, undertaken by a team led by Dr Michael Marcy at the Southern California Evidence-Based Practice Center, estimates that eight children with AOM need to be treated with antibiotics for one child to benefit (Marcy *et al.*, 2001). This estimate is similar to those of earlier reviews, which estimated an NNT of about 7, when the primary outcome measure is the absence of all signs and symptoms of AOM after 7 days of therapy. This means that six out of every seven children with AOM either do not need antibiotics for primary control, or will not respond to antibiotic therapy. All seven children have to be treated, as we cannot predict which of them is at risk for failure. Provided that the antibiotic is safe, well tolerated and affordable, each GP has to decide whether this many children should be treated in order to help a few. Fewer children were still in pain 2 days after treatment with antibiotics started, but the NNT was 21 for this outcome. Fewer children experienced contralateral AOM when treated with antibiotics (NNT = 17).

One of the many formerly accepted ideas about AOM was that very young children were more at risk for serious illness and complications, and would therefore benefit more from antibiotic therapy. The only systematic review to consider treatment for young children, by Dr Roger Damoiseaux of Utrecht University (Damoiseaux *et al.*, 1998) found no difference between antibiotics and placebo.

Another idea that tends to persist is that antibiotics will prevent suppurative complications. The systematic reviews have shown that antibiotic therapy has no effect on recurrent AOM, and offers no protection against hearing loss at 1–2 months post-therapy (Marcy, 2001; Glasziou, 2002). There was a trend towards fewer perforations in the antibiotic-treated group, but the numbers were too small to be statistically significant (acute perforations usually heal well, without hearing loss). Very few serious complications occurred in either the treatment or placebo groups of the many antibiotic trials.

- Amoxycillin remains the recommended first-line therapy.
- Clinical progress is the same when treatment is given for 5 days rather than 10 days.
- The clinical failure rate is slightly higher if the shorter course is used (NNT = 17).
- The relapse rate is slightly higher if the shorter course is used (NNT = 31).

Even if the GP decides that a child does indeed have AOM, and will perhaps benefit from antibiotic therapy, the doctor still has to decide which antibiotic to give, how long to give it for, and whether treatment should be started immediately or delayed for a short time, to see whether the child improves spontaneously.

In England, Dr Paul Little and colleagues conducted a randomised trial of 315 children aged 6 months to 10 years, with a clinical diagnosis of AOM. Half the parents were asked to wait 72 hours after seeing the doctor, and only to use the antibiotic prescription if the child still had pain or fever, or was not getting better. Immediate antibiotic treatment produced significant but small reductions in duration of earache (1.1 day), duration of ear discharge (0.66 day), number of disturbed nights (0.72 days), number of days crying (0.69 days) and doses of paracetamol taken (0.52 teaspoonfuls daily). However, there was no difference in mean pain score, number of episodes of distress, or days absent from school. The findings suggested that there may be a small symptomatic benefit in a few children, who might not get better as quickly without antibiotics. The investigators commented that 'Immediate antibiotic treatment provides some symptomatic relief in the first 24 hours. For children who are not unwell systemically, a wait-and-see approach seems feasible, and acceptable to parents' (Little *et al.*, 2001).

A review (Kozyrskyj *et al.*, 1998) to determine the effectiveness of courses lasting less than 7 days compared with courses longer than 7 days found that treatment failure, relapse or re-infection were significantly more likely to occur in the short term with 5- day courses than with longer courses. However, by 20–30 days there were no significant differences between groups. At various times up to 3 months, outcomes remained similar. The absolute difference in treatment failure suggested that 17–31 children would have to be treated with a longer course of antibiotics, for one child to benefit. It seems best to offer patients the shorter course of antibiotics, with the proviso that they should return if improvement does not occur.

Antibiotics are associated with an increased rate of vomiting, diarrhoea and rashes. A review by Glasziou (2002) estimated that the number needed to harm (NNH) is in the range 12–17. Adverse effects, usually gastrointestinal, are more common when children are given cephalosporins rather than amoxycillin.

Standard-dose amoxycillin three times a day should be considered as first-line oral therapy for low-risk children (those with no exposure to antibiotics in the last 3 months and not attending day-care centres). Higher-risk children should be given a higher dose of amoxycillin. Amoxycillin is the current antibiotic of choice for the following reasons.

- It gives adequate coverage of all the organisms that commonly cause AOM.
- It has the best activity of all the oral ß-lactam agents against penicillin-resistant *Streptococcus pneumoniae*.
- It has excellent middle ear concentration.
- It has relatively few adverse side-effects.
- It has lower potential to induce resistance than some of the newer antibiotics.
- No other agent has been shown to be superior to amoxycillin in antibiotic trials.

The choice of agent when amoxycillin fails remains unclear. In patients who are allergic to penicillin, TMP/SMX has been recommended as the first-line agent. However, because of increasing resistance, erythromycin/SMX may be preferred, especially in children who have attended day-care centres and who have received antibiotics recently.

Non-antibiotic treatment

If treating AOM with antibiotics will have only a modest effect on symptoms, are there other treatments that doctors can recommend? Trials have shown that ibuprofen and paracetamol are equally effective in controlling pain and fever (NNT = 5), but that they do not affect recovery time. Comfort measures for the sick child, such as holding or rocking them, applying warm compresses to the ear, wiping away drainage as it appears, and elevating the head by raising the head of the bed or cot or by using pillows, are supported by the experience and common sense of countless mothers, not by scientific evidence.

Results from the meta-analyses (Marcy 2001; Glasziou 2002) certainly support the decision to withhold antibiotics in selected patients. This decision needs to take into consideration patient history, lifestyle factors, clinical presentation, opportunity for follow-up, and parental receptiveness. When the decision is made to withhold treatment, patients should be followed up and parents educated about the need to return to the doctor if the condition becomes worse.

The best current advice is that the primary healthcare provider should carefully examine the child and, if AOM is thought to be present, explain to the parent that, given the lack of benefit of antibiotics, conservative management – watchful waiting – is the best initial strategy. The GP can either arrange to check the child again in 2–3 days, or give a delayed prescription for antibiotics, which can be used if the child does not improve. If antibiotics are to be used, amoxycillin is still the best first-line treatment. It seems reasonable to prescribe the antibiotic for only 5 days, with the proviso that the child must be checked if there is no obvious improvement during that time. It is also recommended that all children under 5 years who have suffered from AOM should be checked 1–2 months later, to confirm that there is no persistent middle ear effusion. Obviously, older children with risk factors should also be checked.

If recurrent AOM is present (a minimum of three or more episodes of AOM in a 6-month period or during the winter, or four or more episodes in 1 year), a prophylactic antibiotic regimen should be considered following the treatment for the acute episode.

Otitis media with effusion (OME)

Both doctors and parents are concerned about effusion following AOM. Does it need further treatment? Will the child suffer hearing loss? Will the child need an operation? It is important to remember that middle ear effusion is part of AOM. Effusion following an attack of AOM is not indicative of persistent infection, nor is it indicative of treatment failure – it is part of the progression of the disease. The management of OME is controversial, and current data on medical treatments are inconclusive. As it takes 3 months for 90% of children to clear OME completely after an attack of AOM, it seems prudent to wait this long after the acute attack before considering further specific OME treatment. In an extensive review, the US Agency for Healthcare Research and Quality (2002) found that there was no evidence that OME had a long-term effect on expressive or receptive language skills, or on intelligence during the first 3 years of life. There may have been a slight effect on conductive hearing, but this disappeared as the children grew older. There was also no evidence of long-term benefit from treatment of OME with either oral or topical nasal steroids. Therefore these treatments are not recommended at the present time.

Chronic OME may resolve with watchful waiting, but sometimes requires surgical intervention, especially if the child develops signs of hearing loss or of complications. There is no way of predicting which children will require surgical intervention.

Prophylaxis

- Children with recurrent otitis media may benefit from long-term antibiotic therapy (NNT = 9).
- Pneumococcal vaccine may have a modest effect in older children.
- Breastfeeding and avoiding the use of dummies may have some effect.

Despite the best efforts of parents and family doctors, there still seems to be a small group of unfortunate children who experience repeated attacks of AOM and often have persistent middle ear effusion. A systematic review (Williams *et al.*, 1993) found that such children appeared to benefit from long-term prophylactic antibiotic treatment. The risk reduction was quite low, and the NNT was 9. A set of guidelines developed in Norway (Kavaerner and Mair, 1997) suggests that only children who have had three or more episodes of AOM in the past 6 months, or four or more episodes during the past year, should be considered for such treatment. Otitis media prevention measures that should be discussed with parents include breastfeeding, feeding the child upright if he or she is bottle fed, avoiding exposure to tobacco smoke, limiting exposure to other children if possible, and teaching both adults and children careful hand-washing techniques.

A review by Dr Masja Straetemans of Nijmegen University looked at the effects of pneumococcal vaccination in preventing AOM, in trials that included 46 000 children up to 12 years of age (Straetemans *et al.*, 2002). The pneumococcal vaccine had little effect in preventing AOM in healthy children, and only a moderate effect on children with previously documented effects (the AOM rate was reduced by 19%). The authors concluded that 'The evidence does not support wide-scale use of pneumococcal vaccine; the vaccine may be of use in high-risk populations, and ongoing trials will find this out.'

AOM care in different countries

One of the more intriguing phenomena to emerge from the AOM literature is the wide variation that exists in rates of antibiotic prescribing for AOM by GPs from different countries. Wherever you live, you can be sure that GPs in other countries do things slightly differently. The Netherlands has a far lower rate of antibiotic prescribing (and a lower prevalence of resistant strains of bacteria) than other countries, possibly as a result of their guidelines, which strongly emphasise symptomatic treatment and watchful waiting. A cross-national study from GP practice networks in Canada, the Netherlands, the UK and the USA, by Dr Jack Froom and colleagues, found that 97% of North American children were treated with an antimicrobial medication for 10 days, 99% of children in the UK were treated for 5–7 days, but only 17% of children in the Netherlands received a prescription for an antibiotic (Froom *et al.*, 2001). North American doctors were more likely than their UK or Dutch counterparts to prescribe a second-line agent for patients with signs of increased severity. In all three groups, children frequently had an upper respiratory tract infection in the week prior to developing otitis media. The Dutch children had the highest rates of fever, tympanic membrane perforation, otorrhoea and abnormal tympanograms, but even these rates were very low. In addition to the Netherlands, Iceland, Switzerland and Finland have lower antibiotic prescribing rates. No epidemics of sick and deafened children have been reported from the lower-prescribing nations. Thus the evidence supports moderation in antibiotic prescribing.

References

Agency for Healthcare Research and Quality (2002) *Diagnosis, Natural History and Late Effects of Otitis Media with Effusion. Summary. Evidence Report/Technology Assessment Number 55.* AHRQ Publication Number 02-E026. Agency for Healthcare Research and Quality, Rockville, MD.

Alberta Clinical Practice Guidelines Program (2003) *Guidelines for the Diagnosis and Treatment of AOM in Children.* Alberta Clinical Practice Guidelines Program, Edmonton, Alberta.

Damoiseaux RA, Von Balen FA, Hoes AW and de Melker RA (1998) Antibiotic treatment of acute otitis media in children under two years of age: evidence-based? *Brit J Gen Pract.* **48**: 1861–4.

Froom J, Culpepper L, Green LA *et al.* (2001) A cross-national study of acute otitis media: risk factors, severity and treatment at initial visit. Report from the International Primary Care Network (IPCN) and the Ambulatory Sentinel Practice Network (ASPN). *J Am Board Fam Pract.* **14**: 406–17.

Glasziou PP, del Mar CB, Sanders SL and Hayem M (2002) Antibiotics for acute otitis media in children (Cochrane Review). In: *The Cochrane Library. Review CD000219.* Update Software, Oxford.

Gooch WM, Blair E, Puopolo A, Paster RZ, *et al.* (1996) Effectiveness of 5 days of therapy with cefuroxime suspension for the treatment of acute otitis media. *Paediatr Inf Dis J.* **15**: 157–64.

Karma PH, Sipila MM and Kataja MD (1993) Pneumatic otoscopy and otitis media: The value of different TM findings and their combinations. In: DJ Kim, CD Bluestone and JO Klein (eds) *Recent Advances in Otitis Media.* 5th International Symposium. Burlington, Ontario, pp. 41–55.

Kavaerner KJ and Mair IW (1997) Acute and recurrent otitis media: guidelines, treatment and prophylaxis. *Tidskr Nor Laegeforen.* **117**: 4096–8.

Kozyrskyj AL, Hildes-Ripstein GE, Longstaffe LEA *et al.* (2000) Short course antibiotics for acute otitis media (Cochrane Review). In: *The Cochrane Library. Review CD001095.* Update Software, Oxford.

Little P, Gould C, Williamson I *et al.* (2001) Pragmatic randomised controlled trial of two prescribing strategies for childhood acute otitis media. *BMJ.* 322: 336–42.

Marcy M, Takata G, Chan S, Shekelle P, Mason W and Wachsman L (2001) *Management of Acute Otitis Media. Evidence Report/Technology Assessment Number 15.* AHRQ Publication Number 01-E010. Agency for Healthcare Research and Quality, Rockville, MD.

Ruuskanen O, Arola M, Putto-Larila A *et al.* (1989) Acute otitis media and respiratory virus infections. *Pediatr Inf Dis J.* **8**(8): 94–9.

Straetemans M, Sansers E, Veerhoven RH, Schilder AG, Damoiseaux R and Zielhuis G (2002) Pneumococcal vaccines for preventing otitis media (Cochrane Review). In: *The Cochrane Library. Review CD001480.* Update Software, Oxford.

Teele DW, Klein JO and Rosner B (1989) Epidemiology of otitis media during the first seven years in children in greater Boston: A prospective cohort study. *J Infect Dis.* **160**: 83–94.

Uhari M, Mantysaari K and Niemala M (1996) A meta-analytic review of the risk factors for acute otitis media. *Clin Infect Dis.* **22**: 1079–83.

Van Buchem FL, Peeters MF and van't Hof MA (1985) Acute otitis media: a new treatment strategy. *BMJ.* **290**: 1033–7.

Williams RL, Chalmers TC, Stange KC *et al.* (1993) Use of antibiotics in preventing recurrent otitis media and treating otitis media with effusion; a meta analytic attempt to resolve the brouhaha. *JAMA.* **270**: 1344–51.

Chapter 6

Acute sinusitis

Epidemiology and aetiology

> - Sinusitis is one of the 10 commonest diagnoses in primary care.
> - One in 10 people visit their doctor with sinusitis each year.

Approximately 0.5% of all upper respiratory tract infections are complicated by sinusitis, which is one of the most commonly reported respiratory diseases (it is one of the 10 commonest diagnoses in general practice). The incidence of sinusitis ranges from 15 to 43 episodes per 1000 patients per year, depending on the setting (Royal College of GPs, 1986, Hoogen *et al.*, 1985). It is much more common in adults than in children, whose sinuses are not fully developed (Aitken and Taylor, 1992)

> - Most acute sinusitis is caused by virus infections.
> - A small but unknown proportion of cases develop secondary bacterial infection.
> - When sinus aspirates are cultured, most of them are sterile.
> - Figures from ENT clinics which claim that 20–50% of acute sinusitis is bacterial are subject to referral bias. The primary care figure is much lower.

Most acute sinusitis is caused by the same types of viruses that cause the common cold (Gwaltney *et al.*, 1992). A secondary bacterial infection develops in an unknown but small number of cases in primary care. The bacterial pathogens of primary care cases are not really known (culture studies have taken place in specialist and hospital practice) because a sinus puncture to confirm inflammation of the sinus with empyema is hardly ethical and certainly not feasible in general practice. It is estimated that about one-third of adult patients seen in ENT clinics may have acute bacterial rhinosinusitis. Several studies in this referred group of patients have found that in adults, *Streptococcus pneumoniae* and *Haemophilus influenzae* are the commonest bacteria. In the few studies that have been done on children, *Moraxella catarrhalis* has also commonly been found. These are the same bacteria as those associated with acute otitis media. The prevalence of bacterial sinusitis in primary care settings is much lower than in ENT clinic populations, but the exact rate is not known. According to various epidemiological estimates, only 0.2–2% of colds in adults are complicated by bacterial rhinosinusitis (Gwaltney *et al.*, 1992; Puhakka *et al.*, 1998)

Clinical course and management

- Most cases of acute sinusitis will get better without treatment.
- Most patients will be better within 7–10 days.
- When symptoms persist beyond 7 days, bacterial sinusitis is more likely.
- Complications of acute bacterial sinusitis are very rare.

Details of the natural history of the illness have been obtained, as usual, from the placebo-control groups of antibiotic trials. Most adult patients become well or nearly well after 7–10 days, but 25% are still symptomatic after 14 days. Sinusitis sufferers will usually recover spontaneously without antibiotic treatment, even if the infection is bacterial (Stalman *et al.*, 2001). Acute bacterial sinusitis is usually a secondary infection of a common cold, resulting from sinus ostia obstruction and impairment of mucus clearance mechanisms caused by a common cold. The gold standard for bacterial diagnosis is sinus puncture, but because no simple and accurate surgery-based test for acute bacterial sinusitis exists, family doctors rely on clinical findings to make the diagnosis. The signs and symptoms of acute bacterial sinusitis and of a prolonged cough and cold are very similar, which makes diagnosis difficult. Complications are very rare, in both adults and children (none occurred in the placebo arms of all the antibiotic treatment trials in general practice).

Diagnosis of bacterial sinusitis

Many investigators have published reports attempting to identify clinical signs and symptoms specific to acute bacterial rhinosinusitis, to enable GPs to reliably diagnose the condition. All of these studies have had limitations, such as a suboptimal gold standard or variable selection criteria. There are no robust decision rules for bacterial sinusitis, in contrast to the situation for diagnosis of streptococcal sore throat. However, many studies have suggested that the following features are most helpful in predicting the likelihood of bacterial infection following a cold (Alberta Clinical Guidelines, 2000):

1 purulent nasal discharge
2 unilateral maxillary tooth or facial pain, or unilateral sinus tenderness
3 worsening of symptoms after initial improvement
4 lack of response to decongestants.

- Diagnosis is difficult. GPs probably over-diagnose acute sinusitis.
- The best clinical pointers are:
  - previous common cold
  - poor response to decongestants
  - unilateral face or tooth pain, pain on chewing
  - two-phase illness lasting for more than 10 days
  - purulent unilateral nasal discharge
  - tenderness over sinuses.
  If one or two of these pointers are present, sinusitis is unlikely. The presence of four or more indicates that sinusitis is likely.
- Use of tests:
  - nasopharyngeal cultures are not recommended
  - transillumination is of doubtful value
  - plain sinus films are of little value
  - ultrasonography is of moderate value.
- Computed tomography (CT) scans are probably the most reliable test.

Abnormal transillumination, persistence of symptoms for more than 7 days, worsening of pain on postural change or Valsalva manoeuvre, an erythrocyte sedimentation rate (ESR) of >10 mm/hour and elevated levels of C-reactive protein have also been suggested as useful clinical indicators (Lindbaek, 1996; Stalman *et al.*, 2001). Several studies have found that the use of these clinical signs and symptoms will give a diagnostic accuracy similar to that achieved using sinus radiography.

Sinusitis is usually a clinical diagnosis. GPs rarely order diagnostic tests. However, there have been considerable research efforts to determine the best diagnostic test for sinusitis.

Culture

Cultures obtained from the nose or the nasopharynx of patients with acute sinusitis are of no value, as the results do not reflect the pathogenic organism that is causing the sinusitis (Axelsson and Brorson, 1973; Gwaltney *et al.*, 1992).

Transillumination

The value of transillumination of the sinuses is controversial. The sensitivity of transillumination has been found to be limited. Failure to transilluminate does not establish a diagnosis of acute sinusitis. It works better in the hands of expert operators, such as ENT specialists (Low *et al.*, 1997).

X-rays

Sinus X-rays have low sensitivity, and do not distinguish between viral and bacterial sinusitis. The presence of thickened sinus mucosa and fluid levels is more useful for diagnosing chronic rather than acute sinusitis (AHCRP, 1999).

Ultrasonography

Ultrasonography studies have provided varying results, possibly because of differences in patient populations, ultrasonography techniques, or medical personnel involved in testing (Otten *et al.*, 1991; Puhakka *et al.*, 1998). The test is not considered useful for acute sinusitis.

CT scan

CT scanning has been touted by some specialists in the USA as 'a more or less obligatory diagnostic procedure.' CT scans of the sinuses are more sensitive than plain film in identifying sinus infections. However, more than 40% of adults and children undergoing CT scanning for some other reason show some sinus mucosal abnormality (Havas *et al.*, 1988), and up to 87% of adults with early cold symptoms show some sinus abnormalities on CT scan (Gwaltney, 1994). Perhaps the CT scan is most useful for evaluating chronic sinusitis that does not respond to medical treatment, because it will identify anatomical abnormalities and the extent of the disease process.

At present there seems to be no place for routine diagnostic tests for sinusitis in primary care. The development of an evidence-based clinical decision rule would be helpful to GPs.

Treatment: comfort measures

- Most cases of acute sinusitis will recover spontaneously.
- Comfort measures are traditional:
  - inhale steam
  - maintain hydration

> - apply warm facial packs
> - administer saline nasal drops
> - use decongestants
> - sleep with the head of the bed elevated
> - avoid cigarette smoke.
> - There is no convincing evidence that any of these measures are effective.
> - Antihistamines are not recommended.

In primary care, acute sinusitis is mostly a self-limiting disease, so only comfort measures are usually needed. Textbooks discuss the benefits of comfort measures, even though no good-quality studies have been done to quantify their actual effects (Isselbacher *et al.* 1991; Ivker RS, 1995). The following are often suggested:

- maintenance of adequate hydration and inhalation of steam from the bath or shower (to loosen secretions)
- application of warm facial packs (to help to promote drainage of mucus)
- administration of analgesics (for localised pain and tenderness)
- use of saline nose-drop irrigation (to provide moisture and improve mucociliary function).

Adequate rest is advised. Sleeping with the head of the bed elevated is thought to promote sinus drainage. Avoiding cigarette smoke or extremely cool or dry air may prevent dryness and irritation of the mucosa.

No controlled trials have been done to assess the efficacy of decongestants, but numerous authorities recommend them. They are known to increase ostial diameter, and may thus promote sinus drainage. Antihistamines are not recommended, as they cause further inspissation of secretions.

Treatment: antibiotics

> GPs prescribe antibiotics for 77–100% of cases of 'acute sinusitis'
>
> ## In adults
>
> - If acute maxillary sinusitis has been confirmed by radiographs or sinus aspirate:
>   - there is a moderate effect of treatment with penicillin or amoxycillin (NNT = 16)

> – the effect is on purulent sputum rather than on illness symp-
> toms.
> • If acute maxillary sinusitis is diagnosed on clinical grounds there is
> no evidence that antibiotics are of benefit.
> • If antibiotics are used:
> – there is no one best antibiotic; use the cheapest one
> – 10- to 14-day courses are empirically recommended, but shorter
> courses are probably just as effective.
>
> ### In children
>
> • The results of trials (none of which were conducted in primary
> care settings) are controversial.
> • Antibiotics may be helpful for children with persistent nasal
> discharge (NNT = 6).

Only a few good-quality trials of antibiotic treatment have been conducted
in typical primary care settings, for adult patients with sinusitis-like
symptoms. The majority of the trials have shown no effect (American
Academy of Pediatrics, 2001). One or two studies have shown that
antibiotics clear up purulent nasal discharge but have minimal effect on
the duration of illness (Otten and Grote, 1998; Contopoulos-Ioannidis,
2003). Systematic reviews, such as that by Dr John Williams of Duke
University Medical Center in the USA (Williams *et al.*, 2002), have
concluded that the size of the beneficial effects, if any, is probably
clinically non-significant (NNT = 16), and patients on antibiotics are
more likely to develop diarrhoea from the antibiotics than to benefit
from them. Studies of more severely ill patients treated by specialists show
a larger effect, but these results are not applicable to the typical primary
care patient. A couple of small trials have suggested that patients may
benefit from the addition of intranasal steroids to the antibiotic treatment,
but the evidence for this treatment is weak.

Despite the negative (or minimal) results of placebo-controlled trials,
surveys in Denmark, the USA, the UK, the Netherlands, Norway and
France found that more than 90% of patients with a diagnosis of sinusitis
by primary care physicians receive an antibiotic prescription (de Bock *et
al.*, 1997; Bro and Malbeck, 1986; Ferrand *et al.*, 2001). Despite its
predominantly viral aetiology, GPs tend to regard acute sinusitis as a
bacterial disease. 'Sinusitis', like 'bronchitis', seems to be a label that GPs
attach to patients in order to justify their prescription of antibiotics.

It does not appear to matter which antibiotic is used. All of them are
equally effective, and reviews such as that by Dr Donald Low at the

University of Toronto and his colleagues at the Canadian Sinusitis Symposium recommend the use of the cheaper broad-spectrum antibiotics, if antibiotics are used (Low *et al.*, 1997). Although doctors habitually prescribe a 10- or 14-day course of antibiotics, several reviews have suggested that shorter courses may be equally effective (Alberta Clinical Practice Guidelines, 2002; Institute for Clinical Systems Improvement, 2002; Snow *et al.*, 2001).

There are no good-quality primary care studies of antibiotic treatment for sinusitis in children. Because children barely have any sinuses until they are in their teens acute sinusitis is a very rare condition in primary care in this age group. The few trials that do exist were conducted in specialist clinics. They have yielded varying results, and have generated vigorous debate among paediatric ENT specialists about the best management option. The use of antibiotics does appear to clear up purulent nasal discharge (NNT = 6) (American Academy of Pediatrics, 2001) but there is little evidence that the acute illness has a shorter course or is less severe when antibiotics are used in children (Morris and Leach, 2002).

The diagnosis and treatment of acute sinusitis present two of the classic primary care dilemmas – how to diagnose a condition when neither clinical criteria nor tests are perfect, and how to treat the illness when the evidence for effective treatment is weak and contradictory. Because antibiotics can eliminate bacteria, bacterial sinusitis infections need to be identified. At present there is no way of identifying the subgroup of sinusitis patients who are most likely to benefit from antibiotic treatment. And then, which antibiotic should be used? And for how long?

- Wait and see for 7–10 days after initial presentation.
- Tell the patient that they have a 'head cold' rather than 'sinusitis.'
- If symptoms persist, use clinical criteria to diagnose acute sinusitis.
- If a diagnosis is made, prescribe amoxycillin or a folate inhibitor.
- Prescribe antibiotics for 7–10 days.
- Using this strategy will result in a 90% cure rate after 1 week of treatment.

At the prevalence of acute bacterial rhinosinusitis that is likely to be encountered in most primary care settings, the evidence indicates that a strategy of either initial symptomatic treatment or the use of clinical criteria to guide treatment would be an effective and cost-effective approach for uncomplicated patients. A study in the Netherlands by Dr Gert de Bock and colleagues from the University of Leiden (de Bock *et al.* 2001) tested various strategies. 'Wait and see for a week' resulted in 91%

recovery, 'prescribing antibiotics selectively' resulted in 93.2% recovery, and 'prescribing antibiotics immediately' resulted in 94% recovery. Obviously a wait-and-see strategy is most cost-effective.

Several studies have shown that if patients are told that they have 'sinusitis' rather than a 'head cold', and are prescribed antibiotics rather than given advice, they are no more likely to recover quickly, and they become more likely to return to the GP the next time they get a cold.

References

Agency for Healthcare Policy and Research (1999) *Diagnosis and Treatment of Acute Bacterial Rhinosinusitis. Evidence Report/Technology Assessment Number 9.* AHCPR Publication Number 99-E016. Agency for Health Care Policy and Research, Rockville, MD.

Aitken M and Taylor JA (1992) Prevalence of clinical sinusitis in young children followed by primary care physicians. *J Allergy Clin Immunol.* **90**: 433–6.

Alberta Clinical Practice Guidelines Program (2000) *The Diagnosis and Management of Acute Bacterial Sinusitis.* Alberta Clinical Practice Guidelines Program, Edmonton, Alberta.

American Academy of Pediatrics, Subcommittee on Management of Sinusitis and Committee on Quality Improvement (2001) Clinical practice guideline: management of sinusitis. *Pediatrics.* **108**: 798–808.

Axelsson A and Brorson JE (1973) The correlation between bacterial findings in the nose and maxillary sinus in acute maxillary sinusitis. *Laryngoscope.* **83**: 2003–11.

de Bock GH, Dekker FW, Stolk J, Springer MP *et al.* (1997) Antimicrobial treatment in acute maxillary sinusitis: a meta-analysis. *Clin Epidemiology.* **50**: 881–9.

de Bock GH, Van Erkel ER, Springer MP and Kievit J (2001) Antibiotic prescription for acute sinusitis in otherwise healthy adults: clinical cure in relation to costs. *Scand J Primary Health Care.* **19**: 58–63.

Bro F and Malbeck CE (1986) Treatment of infectious diseases in general practice. *Ugeskr Laeger.* **148**: 2540–3.

Contopoulos-Ioannidis DG, Ioannidis JP and Law J (2003) Acute sinusitis in children: current treatment strategies. *Paediatric Drugs.* **5**: 71–80.

Ferrand PA, Mercier PH, Jankowski R *et al.* (2001) Acute sinusitis in adults. Management by general practitioners. *Presse Med.* **30**: 1049–54.

Gwaltney JM, Scheld WM, Sande MA and Sydnor A (1992) The microbial etiology and antimicrobial therapy of adults with acute community-acquired sinusitis: a 15-year experience at the University of Virginia and a review of other selected studies. *J Allergy Clin Immunol.* **90** (Suppl. 3): 457–61.

Gwaltney JM, Phillips R, Miller RD and Riker DK (1994) Computed tomographic study of the common cold. *J Gen Intern Med.* **9**: 38–45.

Havas TE, Morbey JA and Gullane PJ (1988) Prevalence of incidental abnormalities in CT scans of the paranasal sinuses. *Arch Otolaryngol Head Neck Surg.* **114**: 856–9.

Hoogen HJ, Huygen FL, Schellekens JW *et al.* (1985) *Morbidity Figures from General Practice 1978–1982.* Nijmeegs Universitat Huisarten Institut, Nijmegen.

Institute for Clinical Systems Improvement (2002) *Health Care Guideline: acute sinusitis in adults. General implementation*; www.icsi.org

Isselbacher KJ, Braunwald E and Wilson P (1991) In: Harrison *Principle of Internal Medicine* (13e). Lea and Febiger, Malvern, PA. pp. 516–17.

Ivker RS (1995) *Sinus Survival*. GP Putnam's Sons, New York, pp. 67–83.

Lindbaek M, Hjortdahl P and Johnsen U (1996) Use of symptoms, signs and blood tests to diagnose acute sinus infections in primary care: comparison with computed tomography. *Family Practice*. **28**: 183–8.

Low DE, Desrosiers M, McSherry J *et al.* (1997) The Canadian Sinusitis Symposium. A practical guide for the diagnosis and treatment of acute sinusitis. *Can Med Assoc J*. **156 (Suppl. 6)**: S1–14.

Morris P and Leach A (2002) Antibiotics for persistent nasal discharge (rhinosinusitis) in children (Cochrane review). In: *The Cochrane Library CD 001094*. Update Software, Oxford.

Otten FW and Grote JJ (1998) Treatment of chronic maxillary sinusitis in children. *Int J Paedr. Otorhinolaryngology*. **15**: 269–78.

Otten FW, Engberts GE and Grote JJ (1991) Ultrasonography as a method of examination of the frontal sinus. *Clin Otolaryngol*. **16**: 285–7.

Puhakka T, Makela MJ, Alanen K, Kallio T, *et al.* (1998) Sinusitis in the common cold. *J Allergy Clin Immunol*. **102**: 403–8.

Royal College of General Practitioners & DHSS Office of Population Censuses (1986) *Morbidity Statistics from General Practice 1981–1982*. HMSO, London.

Snow V, Mottur-Pilson C and Hickner J (2001) Principles of appropriate antibiotic use for acute sinusitis in adults. *Ann Intern Med*. **34**: 495–7.

Stalman WAB, van Essen GA and van der Graaf Y (2001) Determinants for the course of acute sinusitis in general practice. *Postgrad Med J*. **77**: 778–82.

Williams JW, Aguilar C, Makela M *et al.* (2002) Antibiotics for acute maxillary sinusitis (Cochrane Review). In: *The Cochrane Library. Review CD000243*. Update Software, Oxford.

Chapter 7

Acute bronchitis

Does bronchitis really exist?
Dr William Hueston

Epidemiology and aetiology

- Acute bronchitis is the fifth commonest reason why adults see their GP.
- Around 5% of the adult population seek medical advice for bronchitis each year.
- On average, each attack results in 2–3 days off work.
- Viruses cause 85–95% of cases of acute bronchitis in healthy adults.
- The commonest viruses are rhinovirus, adenovirus, influenza A and B and parainfluenza virus.
- If bacteria are isolated, they may be commensals.
- Bacteria can cause bronchitis in people with underlying health problems. *Mycoplasma pneumoniae, Streptococcus pneumoniae, Haemophilus influenzae, Moraxella catarrhalis* and *Bordetella pertussis* are most commonly involved.

Acute bronchitis is the fifth commonest new problem dealt with by GPs in Australia (Meza *et al.*, 1994) and the USA (Delozier and Gagnon, 1989). It is most common in the 25–65 years age group, and is more frequent in women. In the USA, about 5% of adults self-report an episode of acute bronchitis each year, and up to 90% of them seek medical advice. Population-based estimates of the incidence of acute bronchitis in the UK are 45–50 cases per 1000 people per year. Patients with bronchitis are off work for an average of 2–3 days per episode (McCormick *et al.*, 1995).

It is not easy to isolate micro-organisms from people with acute bronchitis, and microbial studies have only isolated a pathogen in a minority of cases. Respiratory viruses appear to be mainly responsible, causing up to 95% of cases of acute bronchitis in otherwise healthy adults. The commonest viruses are the same as those that cause the common cold, namely rhinovirus, adenovirus, influenza A and B and parainfluenza virus (Verheij *et al.*, 1989; Jonsson *et al.*, 1997).

Even when bacteria have been isolated from sputum samples of people with acute bronchitis, their role is difficult to assess because of the high rates of oropharyngeal colonisation in healthy individuals. Most isolated bacteria are commensals. Bacterial prevalence estimates in cases of acute bronchitis are based on serological criteria because culture of sputum usually yields only commensals, and there is no evidence that these bacteria cause acute bronchitis in adults without underlying lung disease. The commonest non-viral agent is *Mycoplasma pneumoniae*, but *Streptococcus pneumoniae, Haemophilus influenzae, Moraxella catarrhalis* and *Bordetella pertussis* have been implicated in a few cases. *M. pneumoniae* and *Chlamydia pneumoniae* have also been associated with epidemics of bronchitis which occur in the winter, every 4 to 7 years (Jonsson *et al.*, 1997). When bacteria cause acute bronchitis, there is usually some underlying lung disease. Again it is worth noting that the bacteria that have been isolated in bronchitis patients are the same as those which have been implicated in acute sinusitis, pharyngitis and otitis media, thus providing further evidence of the overlapping nature of these ARIs.

Acute bronchitis can also be caused by non-infectious assaults on the bronchial tree by smoke, chemicals and allergens, but these causes are relatively rare.

Clinical course and diagnosis

- The common symptom is an acute cough, which is usually productive. The cough lasts for less than 3 weeks in 50% of patients, but for over 1 month in 25% of patients.
- The appearance of the sputum cannot be used to distinguish between viral and bacterial bronchitis.
- There is no reliable diagnostic sign or laboratory test. The diagnosis is a clinical one.
- There is considerable clinical overlap between acute bronchitis and the other ARIs and pneumonia.
- Results from the control groups of trials show that 85% of patients will improve without specific treatment.

As acute bronchitis is an acute infection of the tracheo-bronchial tree, its hallmark is a cough, which is usually productive. There are transient inflammatory changes in the airways, which produce sputum and symptoms of airways obstruction. The cough commonly lasts for 7–10 days, but may last for up to 3 weeks in 50% of patients and for more than a month in 25% of patients (Hueston and Mainous, 199). The sputum may be either clear or purulent. The appearance of coloured sputum cannot be used to predict whether an infection is viral or bacterial. As with acute sinusitis (*see* Chapter 7), the presence of coloured sputum is due to the release of peroxidases by eosinophilic or neutrophilic leucocytes, and is not caused by the presence of bacteria.

When the clinical course of the control patients in antibiotic trials for acute bronchitis was studied, it was found that 85% of patients improved spontaneously (Alberta Guidelines, 2000).

One reason why bronchitis is such a common diagnosis is that various conditions are often grouped under the heading of bronchitis – the definition is ambiguous. There are no reliable diagnostic signs or laboratory tests, so the diagnosis of acute bronchitis is essentially a clinical one. The most important condition to rule out is acute pneumonia. This can be difficult, as patients with pneumonia and those with bronchitis may both have added lung sounds and fever (unfortunately, these signs are neither sensitive nor specific for pneumonia). Colds and sinusitis can also be confused with acute bronchitis. In both of these illnesses, patients may have a productive cough. A normal lung examination does not rule out acute bronchitis. Bronchitis patients develop a productive cough and often show signs of bronchial obstruction, such as wheezing or dyspnoea on exertion. However, unlike that in asthma, the inflammation in acute bronchitis is transient and usually resolves completely soon after the infection clears up.

Because of the overlap between bronchitis, common cold, sinusitis, asthma and pneumonia, the prevalence estimates usually quoted for bronchitis may be too high. A retrospective chart audit study undertaken by Hueston *et al.* (2000) in the USA compared 135 'acute bronchitis' patients with 409 'upper respiratory tract infection' patients, by looking at a wide variety of patient and doctor characteristics. The study found that there was considerable overlap between the two categories. The strongest positive predictors of acute 'bronchitis' were cough and wheezing on examination. People with a diagnosis of bronchitis were older, and were more likely to be smokers, to have suffered from bronchitis before, to have coughs and wheezes, and (interestingly) to have older doctors. People with 'upper respiratory tract infection' were more likely to have red noses and runny noses, and to experience nausea. Nonetheless, there was considerable overlap of all symptoms and signs, and the investigators commented 'We hypothesise that sinusitis, upper respiratory infection and bronchitis are all variations of the same clinical condition and should be conceptualized as a single clinical entity, with primary symptoms related to different anatomic areas, rather than as different clinical conditions' (Hueston *et al.*, 2000).

A questionnaire study (Oeffinger *et al.*, 1997) of 500 randomly selected American GPs found that, for a diagnosis of acute bronchitis to be made, 58% of GPs said that the cough should be productive, and 60% said that the sputum should be purulent, while 72% felt that wheezing need not be present. Younger physicians and those who prescribed antibiotics as their first choice of treatment were more likely to define acute bronchitis as the presence of purulent sputum.

Using spirometric testing, it has been shown that the signs of acute bronchitis are very similar to those of mild asthma. In one study (Williamson, 1987) forced expiratory volume (FEV1) and peak flow rate (PFR) declined to less than 80% of the predicted values in almost 60% of people with acute bronchitis. Over the 5 weeks following infection these values returned to normal. However, spirometry cannot be used to reliably diagnose acute bronchitis. The situation was further confused by another study (Williams and Schultz, 1989), which found that patients with acute bronchitis were 6.5 times more likely to have been told that they had asthma in the past and 9 times more likely to be diagnosed with asthma in the future. Examination in both conditions may reveal wheezing and a prolonged expiratory phase.

- There is evidence that antibiotics confer minimal benefits on healthy adults with bronchitis:
  - a reduction in duration of cough (NNT = 5)
  - a slightly earlier return to work/normal activities (NNT = 18).
- Antibiotics may have a modest beneficial effect in certain groups of patients, such as older people and those who have been ill for some time. Smokers do not gain any additional benefit from antibiotics.
- Antibiotics cause side-effects (NNH = 14).
- Bronchodilators may help to relieve the cough in people who show evidence of bronchospasm.
- Cough suppressants are of no value for either adults or children.

Treatment of acute bronchitis

Antibiotics

In Australia, it was found that antibiotics were prescribed for acute bronchitis 86% of the time (Meza *et al.*, 1994) whereas in the USA the rate of antibiotic prescribing for acute bronchitis was 60–80% (Mainous *et al.*, 1996). When members of the American Board of Family Practice were questioned (Oeffinger, 1997), 63% of them said that antibiotics were their first choice of treatment for the otherwise healthy, non-smoking adult with acute bronchitis. The decision to use antibiotics as first choice of treatment did not vary with physician's age, gender, number of years in practice, practice type or practice location. The physicians said that they prescribed an antibiotic 75% of the time when they were treating smokers. A survey of GPs in the UK (Stocks and Fahey, 2004) found that 89% would prescribe antibiotics if the sputum was purulent, and that fever and crackles in the chest were the next most important reasons. High levels of antibiotic prescribing are also found among Scandinavian GPs (Straand et al., 1998). Once again, as in the treatment of otitis media, GPs in the Netherlands are the odd men out. A survey of GPs in Holland (Kuyvenhoven et al., 2000) found that they prescribed antimicrobial agents for only 30% of patients with acute bronchitis.

It is likely that these high rates of antibiotic prescribing represent another example of the labelling phenomenon (described in Chapter 7). When GPs have decided to give a coughing patient treatment with antibiotics, they record 'bronchitis' as their preferential diagnosis in the medical record.

Bronchitis does not seem to attract as much research interest as some other ARIs. There have been far fewer trials of antibiotic treatment for acute bronchitis than for AOM or GABHS sore throat. Fortunately, most of the few good-quality trials have been conducted in typical family practice settings in the UK (Howie and Clark, 1970), the USA (Williamson, 1984) and the Netherlands (Verheij et al., 1994). These trials show that acute bronchitis, like sinusitis, is an illness of adults, although it occasionally occurs in adolescents.

Six reviews or critical appraisals of the antibiotic trials for chronic bronchitis have been undertaken. Three reviews found no benefit from using antibiotics (Mackay, 1996; Fahey et al., 1998; Bent et al., 1999). The other three reviews (including one for the Cochrane Collaboration by Dr John Smucny of the University of New York) (Smucny et al., 2004; Orr et al., 1993; Chandran, 2001) found some modest treatment effects when antibiotics were compared with placebo. The use of antibiotics decreased the duration of cough and sputum production by approximately half a day, and time lost from work by 0.3 days. Patients who were taking antibiotics were less likely to report feeling unwell at a follow-up visit, to show no improvement by physician assessment, or to have abnormal lung findings. They also had a slightly shorter duration of coughing and feeling ill (again, about half a day less). There was no difference in sputum production or purulence of sputum, but abnormal lung examinations were less likely in the antibiotic-treated group. Patients who were taking antibiotics used less cough and cold medications. For most of the measures of outcome, the pooled differences were trends, and did not reach the level of statistical significance.

Overall, these reviews estimated that five patients would need to be treated with antibiotics to result in one patient coughing less at follow up, and 18 patients would need to be treated to result in one patient being generally improved. On the other hand, one in 14 patients who were treated with antibiotics experienced adverse side-effects, such as diarrhoea and rashes. The consensus seems to be that antibiotics have a modest benefit, but only for a minority of patients (who cannot easily be identified on presentation to the GP), and that they are therefore not needed to treat most patients with acute bronchitis. Several authors have commented that the beneficial effects of antibiotics may have been overestimated because of publication bias (i.e. the increased tendency to publish studies with significant outcomes). However, the magnitude of any benefit is similar to that of the detriment resulting from potential adverse side-effects. It is also possible that the modest benefits noted were due to the inclusion in some studies of patients who had pneumonia rather than bronchitis, because of the difficulty in discriminating between the two conditions.

In the antibiotic trials amoxycillin, doxycycline, erythromycin and trimethoprim-sulphamethoxazole were used. Any of these seems a reasonable first choice if a family doctor decides to give antibiotics.

Community physicians in the USA prescribe antibiotics to 80–90% of smokers with acute bronchitis. A systematic review was undertaken by Dr Jeffrey Linder, of Massachusetts General Hospital, to determine the efficacy of antibiotics for smokers with acute bronchitis (Linder and Sim, 2002). There have been no studies specifically addressing antibiotic use in smokers, but eight placebo-controlled trials yielded 276 smokers (out of 774 patients). Smoking status did not predict or alter patients' response to antibiotics. The authors concluded that 'The existing evidence suggests that any benefit of antibiotics in smokers is the same as or less than in non-smokers' (Linder and Sim, 2002).

Identification of the few cases of bacterial *Mycoplasma*-associated bronchitis might seem to be a reasonable strategy for selecting patients for whom antibiotic treatment would be beneficial. Unfortunately, there is no clinical method that would enable GPs to distinguish this type of bronchitis. Similarly, it would be helpful to identify cough due to *Bordetella pertussis*, but this is also difficult, unless a local epidemic is in progress or the patient has been exposed to a known index case.

Bronchitis is typically a disease of adults, and only one good-quality trial, conducted by Dr Dana King and colleagues at East Carolina University (King *et al.*, 1996) included some children. A total of 91 American children aged 8 years or over were given erythromycin, 250 mg four times daily for 10 days, or placebo. The children who took antibiotics missed significantly less school, but there were no significant differences in cough, use of cough medicine, general well-being or chest congestion. There is currently no good evidence for treatment of coughing children with antibiotics.

Bronchodilators

As reversible airway obstruction exists in about 50% of patients with acute bronchitis, it seemed reasonable to try bronchodilators as therapy. The evidence for their benefit is conflicting. One review (Williamson, 1987) claimed that randomised controlled trials have demonstrated a consistent benefit from bronchodilator versus placebo, reducing the duration and severity of the cough, with about 50% fewer patients reporting cough after 7 days of treatment (NNT = 4). A systematic review (Smucny *et al.*, 2004) disagreed with these findings, and concluded that although some individual trials appeared to show benefit, overall there were no significant benefits. There were no significant differences in daily cough scores or in the number of patients still coughing after 7 days, and patients were much more likely to report side-effects such as tremor, shakiness or nervousness (NNH = 2.3). There is little evidence to support the routine use of beta-agonists for adults who have acute cough, unless there is evidence of airflow obstruction, in which case these agents may reduce symptoms, including cough.

Cough medicines

Non-specific cough therapy is commonly prescribed to patients either together with or in lieu of antibiotics. An older review, by Dr Richard Irwin of the University of Massachusetts Medical School (Irwin and Curley, 1991), found limited evidence to support the use of codeine and dextromorphan in some patients. The literature evaluating the efficacy of antitussive therapy is problematic because treatment benefit appears to depend on the cause of the cough. Acute coughs due to colds do not appear to respond to dextromorphan or codeine, whereas chronic cough due to underlying lung disease seems to respond to some degree to these two agents. Once again it is a judgement call for the GP. A recent evidence-based guideline from the American College of Chest Physicians (2006) recommends that 'Antitussive agents are occasionally useful, and can be offered for short-term symptomatic relief of coughing.' This report strongly suggests that over-the-counter cough medicines should not be given to children, because of their potential side-effects.

Current evidence supports the need to minimise antibiotic prescribing for patients with uncomplicated acute bronchitis. The modest benefits need to be weighed against the harmful side-effects. Further studies are needed to identify the particular subsets, if any, of coughing patients who may benefit from antibiotics. Until further well-controlled clinical trials have been conducted, bronchodilators should only be used if the patient has abnormal findings on lung examination, or exhibits clinical wheezing and a tight cough. Symptomatic treatments that may help people with acute bronchitis include hydration, bed rest, and relief of pain and fever. A cough suppressant may help a non-productive cough in some patients.

Patients should be given a realistic prediction of the duration of their cough, which will typically last for at least 10–14 days after the surgery visit. Doctors might consider calling the cough a 'chest cold' rather than 'acute bronchitis.' Use of the term 'chest cold' in the USA was associated with much less frequent belief that antibiotic therapy was needed (King *et al.*, 1996). Patients could be told that antibiotic use will increase the likelihood of their carrying resistant organisms, and that antibiotics commonly have side-effects. Clinicians caring for patients with uncomplicated acute bronchitis should be encouraged to discuss the lack of benefit of antibiotic treatment for the condition, and stop prescribing antibiotics.

References

Alberta Clinical Guidelines Program (2000) *Guideline for the Management and Treatment of Acute Bronchitis.* Alberta Clinical Guidelines Program, Edmonton, Alberta.

American College of Chest Physicians (2006) Diagnosis and management of cough: executive summary. ACCP evidence-based clinical practice guidelines. *Chest.* **129**: 1–23S.

Bent S, Saint S, Itinghoff E and Grady B (1999) Antibiotics in acute bronchitis: a meta-analysis. *Am J Med.* **107**: 62–7.

Chandran R (2001) Should we prescribe antibiotics for acute bronchitis? *Am Fam Physician.* **64**: 135–8.

Delozier JE and Gagnon RO (1989) *National Ambulatory Care Survey 1989 Summary: Advance data.* National Center for Health Statistics, Hyattsville, MD. Pub No. 203.

Fahey T, Stocks N and Thomas R (1998) Quantitative systematic review of randomised controlled trials comparing antibiotic with placebo for acute cough in adults. *BMJ.* **316**: 906–10.

Hueston WJ and Mainous AG (1998) Acute bronchitis. *Am Fam Physician.* **57**: 1270–82.

Hueston WJ, Mainous AG, Dacus EN and Hopper JE (2000) Does acute bronchitis really exist? A reconceptualization of acute viral respiratory tract infection. *J Fam Pract.* **49**: 401–6.

Howie JG and Clark GA (1970) Double-blind trial of early dimethylchlortetracycline in minor respiratory illness in general practice. *Lancet.* **2**: 1099–102.

Irwin RS and Curley FS (1991) The treatment of cough: a comprehensive review. *Chest.* **99**: 1477–84.

Jonsson JS, Sigurdsson JA, Kristinsson KG, Guonadottir M and Magnusson S (1997) Acute bronchitis in adults: how close do we come to its aetiology in general practice? *Scand J Prim Health Care.* **15**: 156–60.

King DE, Williams WC, Bishop L and Shecter A (1996) Effectiveness of erythromycin in the treatment of acute bronchitis. *J Fam Practice.* **42**: 601–5.

Kuyvenhoven MM, Verheij TJ, de Melker RA and van der Velden J (2000) Antimicrobial agents in lower respiratory tract infections in Dutch general practice. *Br J Gen Pract.* **50**: 133–4.

Linder JA and Sim I (2002) Antibiotic treatment of acute bronchitis in smokers: a systematic review. *J Gen Intern Med.* **17**: 230–34.

Mackay DN (1996) Treatment of acute bronchitis in adults without underlying lung disease. *J Gen Intern Med.* **11**(9): 557–62.

McCormick A, Fleming D and Charlton J (1995) *Morbidity statistics from general practice. 4th National Morbibity Survey, 1991–1992.* HMSO/Office for National Statistics, London.

Mainous AG, Zoorob RJ and Hueston WJ (1996) Current management of acute bronchitis in ambulatory care. *Arch Fam Med.* **5**: 79–83.

Meza RA, Bridges-Webb C, Sayer GP, *et al.* (1994) The management of acute bronchitis in general practice: results from the Australian Morbidity and Treatment Survey 1990–1991. *Aust Fam Physician.* **23**: 1550–3.

Oeffinger KC, Snell LM, Foster BM, *et al.* (1997) Diagnosis of acute bronchitis in adults: a national survey of family physicians. *J Fam Pract.* **45**: 336–7.

Orr PH, Scherer K, MacDonald A and Moffatt ME (1993) Randomized placebo-controlled trials of antibiotics for acute bronchitis: a critical review of the literature. *J Fam Pract.* **36**: 507–12.

Smucny J, Fahey T, Becker L and Glazier R (2002) Antibiotics for acute bronchitis (Cochrane Review). In: *The Cochrane Library. Review CD000245.* Update Software, Oxford.

Stocks NP and Fahey T (2004) The treatment of acute bronchitis by general practitioners in the UK. Results of a cross-sectional postal survey. *Aust Fam Physician.* **31**: 675–9.

Straand J, Skinio Rostad K and Sandvik H (1998) Prescribing systemic antibiotics in general practice: a report from the More & Romsdal Prescription Study. *Scan J Primary Health Care.* **16**: 121–7.

Williams H and Schultz P (1987) An association between acute bronchitis and asthma. *J Fam Pract.* **24**: 35–8.

Williamson HA (1984) A randomised controlled trial of doxycycline in the treatment of acute bronchitis. *J Fam Pract.* **19**: 481–6.

Williamson H (1987) Pulmonary function tests in acute bronchitis: evidence for reversible airways obstruction. *J Fam Pract.* **25**: 251–6.

Verheij TJ, Kaptein AA and Mulder JD (1989) Acute bronchitis: aetiology, symptoms and treatment. *Fam Pract.* **6**: 66–9.

Verheij TJ, Hermans J and Mulder JD (1994) Effects of doxycycline in patients with acute cough and purulent sputum: a double-blind placebo-controlled trial. *Br J Gen Pract.* **44**: 400–4.

Chapter 8

Influenza

Coughs and sneezes spread diseases.
British World War Two public health slogan

Epidemiology and aetiology

- Up to 20% of the general population are exposed to influenza each year, but only about 10% have a clinical illness, and most do not go to see their GP.
- The incidence of influenza is highest in the winter months.
- The influenza virus is spread by coughing and sneezing.
- Serious illness, excess hospitalisation and death due to influenza occur:
  - in very young children
  - in people aged 65 years or older
  - in people with pre-existing heart or lung diseases.

Influenza is a common acute respiratory illness that may affect up to 20% of the general population annually, although only a small proportion consult the doctor about their clinical symptoms (Couch, 1993). The rates of serious illness, hospitalisation and death are highest among people aged 65 years or over, in young children and in individuals of any age who have medical conditions that place them at increased risk of complications of influenza. People with chronic cardiac and respiratory problems are more likely to be hospitalised or to die as a result of influenza. Other factors associated with poor outcomes are previous hospitalisation, high GP visiting rate and polypharmacy (in other words, people who are already sick and visiting doctors often).

The excess illness burden caused by influenza is high. In the UK, it is associated with 3000 excess deaths/year in non-epidemic years, and with 18 000 deaths/year when there is an epidemic (Ashley *et al.*, 1991). A similar phenomenon has been observed in the US, where influenza epidemics have caused 114 000 excess hospitalisations and 20 000 extra deaths per year (Housworth and Langmuir, 1974).

The influenza virus is spread from person to person primarily by droplet infection. Your mother was right – coughs and sneezes do spread diseases. The virus can survive for up to 48 hours outside the body, on hands, doorknobs and handrails, for example. Influenza viruses cause illnesses among all age groups, but the rates of infection are highest among children. The incubation period is 1–4 days, with an average of 2 days. Adults and children are infectious from the day before symptoms begin until about 5 days after the onset of illness. Severely immunocompromised individuals can shed the virus for weeks. The percentage of infections resulting in clinical illness can range from 10–85%, depending on the patient's age and pre-existing immunity to the virus. Serological conversion to the current influenza strain occurs in 10–20% of the population each year, with the highest rates being seen in those under 20 years of age. The attack rates are higher in institutions such as schools and nursing homes (Harpur, *et al.* 2005).

- The illness is caused by infection with influenza A and B viruses.
- Each year, new variants result from antigen shift. Influenza A changes more often and more quickly than influenza B.

Influenza A and B viruses are the two types of virus that cause epidemic human disease. New influenza virus variants result from frequent antigenic change due to point mutations that occur during viral replication. Influenza A viruses undergo antigenic change more often and more quickly than influenza B viruses. A person's immunity to the surface antigens, especially haemagglutinin, reduces the likelihood and severity of infection. Antibody against one virus or subtype confers limited or no protection against others. Frequent virus variation through antigenic shift is the virological basis for seasonal epidemics, and is the reason why one or more new strains are incorporated in each year's new influenza virus (Kilbourne, 1987).

Clinical course and diagnosis

- The diagnosis is usually clinical, using constitutional symptoms (headache, fever, malaise and myalgia) and respiratory symptoms (cough, sore throat and runny nose).
- The most useful symptoms are sudden onset, fever at onset,

> headache at onset and cough. These can have a positive predictive value of up to 75%.
> * Polymerase chain reaction (PCR) tests can provide a result within 30 minutes, and are 85–95% sensitive.
> * The acute illness lasts for about 3 days, but cough and malaise can persist for weeks.

Influenza infection can be subclinical, producing no illness. In studies of people with the common cold and with bronchitis, influenza viruses are frequently isolated. Respiratory illness caused by influenza is difficult to distinguish from illness caused by other respiratory pathogens. The typical symptoms of influenza are an abrupt onset of constitutional and respiratory signs and symptoms (fever, myalgia, headache, malaise, sore throat and rhinitis). The illness typically resolves after 2–4 days (mean duration of acute illness is 3 days) in most individuals, although cough and malaise can persist for over 2 weeks.

GPs rely on their clinical judgement to diagnose influenza. A study in the Netherlands by Dr Leontine van Elden and colleagues (van Elden *et al.*, 2001) assessed the value of clinical symptoms for diagnosing influenza. They identified patients with a fever and at least one constitutional symptom and one respiratory symptom. They then performed a polymerase chain reaction (PCR) test for influenza on nose and throat swabs. The combination of headache at onset, feverishness at onset and cough had a positive predictive value of up to 75%. Other studies have reported quite high sensitivities and specificities for clinical definitions of influenza (Boivin *et al.*, 2000; Monto *et al.*, 2000). As yet there is no scientifically derived and validated diagnostic decision rule for influenza.

Laboratory tests available for influenza include viral culture, serology, rapid antigen testing, PCR and immunofluorescence tests. Nasopharyngeal specimens are better than throat swabs for isolation and culturing of viruses.

Because the appropriate treatment of patients with influenza depends upon accurate and timely diagnosis, there has been much interest in developing rapid tests for the illness. Several commercial rapid PCR tests are available, but unfortunately they still need to be performed in a laboratory rather than in the doctor's surgery, unlike the rapid GABHS tests for sore throat. These tests can detect influenza viruses within 30 minutes. Some tests detect only influenza A virus, while others detect A and B. The rapid tests have lower sensitivity than viral culture and serology (Cox and Subbarao, 1999). However, a study in Scottish general practice, conducted by Dr William Carman from the Regional Virology Laboratory in Glasgow (Carman *et al.*, 2000) which compared PCR with culture-confirmed influenza, found that the rapid test had only 58% sensitivity. However, PCR did not give any false-positive results, and it was suggested that the rapid, user-friendly test would be useful early in the season to confirm that true influenza was present in the community.

Treatment

There is no role for antibiotics in the treatment of influenza, but GPs often prescribe them for patients with feverish flu-type illnesses, perhaps in the hope of preventing complications.

- Amantidine and rimantidine are effective against influenza A virus only. They can cause transient neurological (NNH ~45) and gastrointestinal (NNH *c*.27) side-effects.
- Zanamivir and oseltamivir work against both influenza A and B viruses. They can cause bronchospasm (NNH *c*.13) and intestinal upsets (NNH *c*.10).
- These drugs must be started within 1–2 days of the onset of illness.
- They reduce illness duration by 1 day and time off work by half a day.
- They have a modest preventive effect on serious complications.

Traditionally, the treatment of influenza always consisted of relief of symptoms and support of the patient by their family. The development of two classes of antiviral agents specifically for influenza has led to suggested changes in management of the situation during influenza epidemics, especially for those who, by virtue of previous illness or occupational hazard, are more likely to contract the illness.

M2 ion-channel blockers

Amantidine and rimantidine are M2 ion-channel blockers (also known as amantadanes), which are specific inhibitors of influenza A virus – they do not work against influenza B viruses. Amantidine-resistant viruses are cross-resistant to rimantidine, and vice versa (Shekel, 1992). These drugs can cause side-effects in the nervous system, such as nervousness, anxiety, insomnia and difficulty concentrating (NNH *c*.45), and in the gastrointestinal tract, such as nausea and anorexia (NNH *c*.27). However, these side-effects are usually mild and cease when the drug is stopped (Soo, 1989).

The neuraminidase inhibitors (NAIs)

Zanamivir and oseltamivir inhibit both influenza A and B viruses. Zanamivir can cause bronchospasm with a decline in FEV1 (NNH = 13) (Jefferson, 2000), so it is not generally recommended for people with underlying respiratory disease. It has to be given by nasal spray, and has been superseded in the market by the orally administered oseltamivir. Nausea and vomiting have been reported in around 10% of patients taking oseltamivir.

When administered within 2 days of the onset of illness in otherwise healthy adults, amantidine and rimantidine can reduce the duration of uncomplicated influenza A illness by about 1 day (from 4 days to 3 days). Zanamivir and oseltamivir can produce a similar reduction in uncomplicated influenza A and B illness, and some studies suggest that the effect can be even stronger if the drug is given very early in the illness (Jefferson, 2001). Even when people are exhibiting symptoms of influenza, zanamivir has been shown to reduce temperature, decrease cough and reduce viral load, so that the patient is less infective. A review of studies conducted in Europe and the USA (Jefferson, 2000) found that people who take oseltamivir are only about half as likely to get influenza, and that the drug can be used to prevent the spread of infection within families and institutions. In addition, the incidence of secondary complications such as pneumonia, bronchitis, sinusitis and otitis media was reduced from 15% to about 8% (NNT = 14).

Prevention of influenza by vaccination

Vaccination is the main mode of influenza prevention. Vaccine can be administered as a live attenuated or inactivated aerosol, or as an inactivated intramuscular injection. It is most often given as a trivalent inactivated preparation which contains the two influenza A viruses and one influenza B virus which have most recently been prevalent in the community. The effectiveness of the vaccine depends largely on the amount of viral antigenic shift that has occurred since the last influenza season, and is also dependent on the age and immunocompetence of the recipient. When the vaccine and the circulating viruses are antigenically similar, influenza vaccination prevents influenza illness in 70–90% of healthy adults (Harpur, *et al.* 2005). Vaccination has also been shown to result in decreased work absenteeism, reduced otitis media in children, a decrease in use of healthcare resources and a reduction in use of antibiotics (Demicheli, 2004).

Because rates of serious illness and death are highest among people over 65 years of age and individuals of any age who have medical conditions

---

- Vaccines usually contain two influenza A inactivated viruses and one influenza B inactivated virus.
- Serious side-effects are very rare.
- Vaccines are 70–90% effective in healthy adults, and 30–70% effective in older and ill people.
- Vaccination is recommended for people aged 65 years or over, children aged 6–23 months, people with chronic cardiac, pulmonary and metabolic conditions, and healthcare workers in long-term care institutions.
- In most countries, the vaccination of healthy adults is not recommended.
- Vaccination has been associated with decreased levels of serious illness, less hospitalisation, fewer deaths, fewer visits to doctors and less time off work.
- Vaccination should take place in the late autumn, but high-risk individuals may be vaccinated even after an influenza epidemic has started.

---

that put them at risk of the complications of influenza, these people are the primary targets for immunisation. Other target groups include individuals who care for or live with people at high risk, such as healthcare workers and family members. The optimal time for vaccination is during October and November (in the Northern hemisphere). Vaccination should continue into December and later, for as long as vaccine is available (Public Health Agency of Canada, 2004). Because very young otherwise healthy children are at risk for influenza-related hospitalisation, vaccination of healthy children aged 6–23 months is encouraged in the USA. Several cost–benefit analyses have found that vaccination produces overall societal cost savings (Centre for Reviews and Dissemination, 1996).

Older people and individuals with chronic diseases develop lower post-vaccination antibody levels than do healthy young adults, and may therefore remain more susceptible to influenza. Trials have shown that vaccine efficacy is lower in older people, especially those who live in nursing homes or similar long-term care facilities. In such settings, influenza vaccine is only 30–60% effective, but is still worthwhile, as it prevents hospitalisation and some deaths (Centre for Reviews and Dissemination, 1996). Vaccination rates in the elderly are increasing. Among people aged over 65 years in the USA, influenza vaccination levels increased from 33% in 1989 to 66% in 1999 (Harpur, *et al.* 2005). Similar improvements have been reported in vaccination rates among nursing home residents, which increased from 64% in 1989 to 83% in 1999 (Gross *et al.*, 1995). There is concern that reported rates of vaccination in at-risk children are very low, and among healthcare workers, low vaccination rates of 34% and 38% were reported in 1999 and 2000, respectively (Harpur, *et al.* 2005). Vaccinating young people works – the majority of children and young adults develop high post-vaccination antibody titres, and the inactivated vaccine is 80–90% effective against influenza respiratory illness (Briss *et al.*, 2000). People at high risk for the complications of influenza can still be vaccinated after an outbreak of flu has begun in their community. The development of antibodies can take up to 2 weeks.

Primary care physicians should emphasise to their patients that inactivated influenza virus vaccine contains killed viruses and cannot cause influenza, and coincidental respiratory disease unrelated to influenza can occur after vaccination. The vaccination will not prevent coughs and colds.

Vaccines do have some side-effects. In placebo-controlled studies of vaccinated adults, the most frequent side-effect was soreness at the vaccination site (in 10–30% of patients) that lasted for less than two days (Briss *et al.*, 2000; Harpur, *et al.* 2005). Fever, malaise and myalgia can occur after vaccination, and most often occur in people who have had no previous exposure to vaccine. These reactions begin 6–12 hours after vaccination and can persist for 1–2 days. Split-virus vaccines have fewer side-effects than whole-virus vaccines. Reviews of trials that included tens of thousands of patients found that serious complications were very rare (Jefferson, 2000).

Vaccines for healthy people

Several systematic reviews of randomised and quasi-randomised trials have examined the impact of vaccination on healthy people. Inactivated parenterally administered vaccines can reduce the incidence of serologically confirmed influenza A by about two-thirds. More importantly, the vaccine was less effective in reducing clinical influenza cases, by only 25% (Demicheli *et al.*, 2004). Although trials consistently show fewer days off work, the reduction is only about half a day. Originally, this modest benefit discouraged the use of vaccination in healthy adults, but recently some jurisdictions, such as the Canadian province of Ontario, have advocated universal vaccination as a public health measure to promote mass immunity. It is too early to judge whether or not this is an effective strategy. Kawaura, a rural town in Japan with a population of 6800, started a mass influenza vaccination in the 1999–2000 season, for all residents over 2 years of age. That year, the relative risk of vaccinated individuals being hospitalised due to respiratory disease was 0.13, and the relative risk for death of vaccinated individuals was 0.28 (Takahashi *et al.*, 2001). Cost-effectiveness studies have suggested that universal vaccination of healthy adults is likely to be more beneficial than offering antiviral therapy to those who become ill, but few countries have adopted such a policy.

The highest rates of infection with influenza virus occur in very young children because of their lack of prior immunity and previous exposure to the virus. Studies of schoolchildren in the USA have shown that they benefit from vaccination. The USA is currently the only developed country that recommends universal influenza vaccination for children aged 6–23 months. In Japan, where childhood mortality from influenza was higher than in the USA or Europe, all schoolchildren were vaccinated against influenza in the years 1962–87. The excess mortality rate dropped to one-third during the vaccination programme, and vaccination prevented an estimated 4000 deaths per year (NNT = 420) (Gruber *et al.*, 1990). After 1987, when the programme stopped, the mortality rate rose to its previous level.

Vaccines for the elderly

Most deaths related to influenza occur in people aged over 65 years, and those with chronic underlying health problems are most at risk. Annual vaccination of older people is a cost-effective way of reducing influenza-related deaths and illnesses. Two meta-analyses have been done on the studies of vaccination effectiveness in the elderly. Vaccination was found to be 56% effective in preventing respiratory illness (NNT *c.2*), 53% effective in preventing pneumonia (NNT *c.2*), 48% effective in preventing hospitalisation (NNT *c.2*) and 68% effective in preventing mortality (NNT *c.1.5*) (Strassburg *et al.*, 1986; Gross *et al.*, 1995). The reviewers cautioned that as most of the studies were non-experimental in design (they were mainly cohort studies), the effectiveness might have been slightly exaggerated, but there is now a large body of evidence which affirms that influenza vaccination does reduce the risk of hospitalisation, pneumonia and mortality in the elderly during an influenza epidemic. It is one of the most efficacious interventions in modern medicine.

Despite publicity campaigns and strong evidence of effectiveness, not all elderly people take the influenza vaccine. A general practice study conducted by Dr Gerrit van Essen in Utrecht in the Netherlands (van Essen, 1997) tried to assess why healthy elderly people failed to comply with influenza vaccination. A survey of non-compliant patients over 65 years of age found that concerns about the side-effects of the vaccine, perceived good health and belief that they were not susceptible to influenza were the commonest reasons for non-compliance.

Vaccines for healthcare workers

There have been several studies, but no systematic reviews, of the effects of vaccinating workers in long-term care hospitals in the USA. Uptake of vaccine was much higher in sites where it was routinely offered to workers, rather than being left to their own discretion. The mortality rate of elderly patients was lower in hospitals where staff had been offered vaccine. One study found that there was one less death for every 11–14 staff members vaccinated (Stott *et al.*, 1997). In 1999, the rate of influenza vaccination among healthcare workers in the USA was only 38%, despite the fact that vaccination was associated with fewer patient deaths and a reduction in the number of days off work (Wilde *et al.*, 1999).

Vaccines for diabetics

Although there have been few clinical trials of vaccine efficacy specifically in patients with diabetes, the Advisory Committee on Immunization Practices in the USA feels that subgroup analysis of the patients with diabetes in large completed cohort and case–control studies supports influenza vaccination in all people with diabetes over 6 months old (Harpur, *et al.* 2005).

Vaccines and lung disease

A prospective cohort study of 1969 patients with chronic lung disease over 18 years of age (mostly with chronic obstructive pulmonary disease and asthma), conducted in general practice settings in the Netherlands by Dr Eelko Hak and his colleagues (Hak *et al.*, 1998) found no effectiveness of the immunisation programme for people aged 18–64 years, whereas in those aged over 64 years the occurrence of any complication was reduced by 50%. Viral respiratory tract infections in patients with cystic fibrosis (CF) cause deterioration of lung function and disease progression. Annual influenza vaccination for these individuals is recommended by the British Joint Committee on Vaccination and Immunisation (JCVI, 1996) although a Cochrane Review by Dr Agnes Tan of the Royal Women's Hospital in Melbourne found that to date no studies have compared vaccine with placebo in this population, and consequently 'There is currently no evidence from randomised studies that influenza vaccine given to patients with CF is of benefit to them' (Tan *et al.*, 2002).

Influenza causes excess hospitalisations in people with asthma, especially children. Vaccination may reduce morbidity in asthmatic infants and preschool children. A retrospective cohort study of 349 children, also conducted by the Utrecht Family Medicine Group (Smits *et al.*, 2002) assessed the effectiveness of trivalent influenza vaccine over two influenza seasons in primary care settings in the Netherlands. Overall, respiratory disease in asthmatic children was reduced by 27%, but in children under 6 years of age the effectiveness was higher, at 55%. Although influenza vaccination is recommended in many countries for people with asthma, there is still a little controversy about administering influenza vaccine, as its use may precipitate an asthma attack in some individuals. For this reason, some physicians still caution against its use. A Cochrane Review by Dr Christopher Cates, a GP from the UK, concluded that there is currently not enough evidence, even from randomised controlled trials, to assess whether influenza vaccine has a protective effect for people with asthma: 'There is a need for larger randomised placebo-controlled trials to determine both the protective and adverse effects of influenza vaccine on ambulatory adults and children with asthma' (Cates *et al.*, 2000).

Improving vaccine uptake

There is little doubt that influenza vaccination is one of the most effective interventions that family doctors can offer their patients. How can we ensure that most or more of the patients who will benefit actually get their vaccine? Various attempts have been made to improve vaccination rates. Reviews of these suggest that multiple methods should be tried (Sarnoff and Rundell, 1999). Patients can be helped by being reminded of the vaccination, and being vaccinated in their own homes if necessary, and the vaccine should be provided free of charge. Vaccine providers should leave standing orders for certain patients, and there should be office or surgery systems that remind providers to give the vaccine. As vaccine uptake rates increase, more complex strategies will be needed to give vaccines to the unvaccinated minority. Organisational changes may be needed to increase the probability of patient–provider contact during the flu season. Possible strategies include walk-in clinics, satellite vaccination sites, or the scheduling of annual physical examinations during the flu season. Two studies in the Netherlands used a computerised reminder system which identified high-risk patients and sent them personal reminders by mail. As a result, vaccine uptake by high-risk patients increased from 40% to 77% (Hak *et al.*, 2002).

Use of antiviral drugs for influenza prevention

In addition to the use of the neuraminidase inhibitors to treat people who have influenza, there has been interest in their protective effect, both for immediate family contacts during individual cases, and for population protection during epidemics. Both rimantidine and oseltamivir have been approved for prophylactic treatment. A systematic review by Matheson *et al.* (2003) examined the prophylactic trials that have been done, and found that as a preventive measure the neuraminidase inhibitors were 74% effective for naturally occurring cases of clinically defined influenza in adults, and 60% effective for laboratory-confirmed influenza. Nursing home studies have found that both amantidine and rimantidine are 70–90% effective in preventing influenza A illness, and can limit the spread of influenza (Sarnoff and Rundell, 1999). Of course, they are ineffective again influenza B illness. Both agents have also been reported to prevent influenza illness among household contacts of influenza cases. Community studies of healthy adults have indicated that both zanamivir and oseltamivir are about 80% effective in preventing febrile, laboratory-confirmed influenza (Matheson *et al.*, 2003).

To be maximally effective as chemoprophylaxis, these drugs must be taken each day for the duration of influenza activity in the community. In practice, they are usually only given during the period of peak activity, which may limit their effect slightly.

Although studies have found that sickness and time off work are reduced in healthcare workers who have been vaccinated, there have been no studies of the effects of chemoprophylaxis for healthcare workers, especially during an epidemic.

Other preventive measures

Transmission can be reduced if influenza sufferers are isolated. The use of masks and of alcohol gels for hand washing has been shown to reduce infection rates.

Pandemic strategies

Since the advent of avian influenza in Asia, and the reports of some human victims, many countries are grappling with the potential problems that will arise if an influenza pandemic ever occurs. Most countries, even in the developed world, do not have plans in place to cope with such a situation. Since 2004, Canada has had a Pandemic Influenza Plan, which involves increasing influenza surveillance systems, upgrading the capacity and speed of response of vaccine manufacture, and stockpiling of antiviral medications (Public Health Agency of Canada, 2004).

References

Ashley J, Smith T and Dunnell K (1991) Deaths in Great Britain associated with the influenza epidemic of 1989–90. *Population Trends*. **62**: 16–20.

Boivin G, Hardy I, Tellier G and Maziade J (2000) Predicting influenza infections during epidemics with use of a clinical case definition. *Clin Infect Dis*. **31**: 1166–9.

Briss PA, Rodewald LE, Hinman AR *et al.* (2000) Reviews of evidence regarding interventions to improve vaccination coverage in children, adolescents and adults. *Am J Prev Med.* **18 (Suppl.):** 97–140.

Carman WF, Wallace LA, Walker J *et al.* (2000) Rapid virological surveillance of community influenza infection in general practice. *BMJ.* **321:** 736–7.

Cates CJ, Jefferson TO, Bara AI and Rowe BH (2000) Vaccines for preventing influenza in people with asthma (Cochrane Review). In: *The Cochrane Library. Review CD000364.* Update Software, Oxford.

Centre for Reviews and Dissemination, University of York (1996) *Effectiveness Matters: Influenza vaccination and older people.* Centre for Reviews and Dissemination, University of York, York.

Couch RB (1993) Advances in influenza virus research. *Annals NY Acad Science.* **605:** 803–12.

Cox MJ and Subbarao K (1999) Influenza. *Lancet.* **354:** 1277–82.

Demicheli V, Rivetti D, Deeks JJ and Jefferson TO (2004) Vaccines for preventing influenza in healthy adults (Cochrane Review). In: *The Cochrane Library. Review CD001269.* Update Software, Oxford.

Gross PA, Hermogenes AW, Sachs HS *et al.* (1995) The efficacy of influenza vaccines in the elderly: a meta-analysis and review of the literature. *Ann Intern Med.* **123:** 518–27.

Gruber WC, Taber LH, Glezen WP *et al.* (1990) Live attenuated and inactivated influenza vaccine in school-age children. *Am J Dis Child.* **144:** 585–600.

Hak E, Nordin J and Wei F (2002) Influence of high-risk medical conditions on the effectiveness of influenza vaccination of the elderly. *Clin Inf Dis.* **35:** 370–7.

Hak E, van Essen G, Buskens E *et al.* (1998) Is immunizing all patients with chronic lung disease in the community against influenza cost effective? *J Epidemiol Comm Health.* **52:** 120–5.

Harpur SA, Fukuda A, Uyeki TM, *et al.* (2005) *Prevention and Control of Influenza:* Recommendations of the Advisory Committee of Immunization Practices (ACIP). MMWR Remomm Rep 54 (RR-8): 1–40.

Housworth J and Langmuir AD (1974) Excess mortality from influenza epidemics, 1957–1966. *Am J Epidemiol.* **100:** 40–8.

Jefferson T, Demicheli V, Deeks J and Rivetti D (2000) Neuraminidase inhibitors for preventing and treating influenza in healthy adults (Cochrane Review). In: *The Cochrane Library. Review CD000269.* Update Software, Oxford.

Joint Committee on Vaccination and Immunization (1996) *Immunization Against Infectious Disease.* HMSO. **113:** 20.

Kilbourne ED (1987) *Influenza.* Plenum Book Co., New York

Matheson NJ, Symmonds-Abraham M, Sheikh A, Sheppard S and Harnden A (2003) Neuraminidase inhibitors for preventing and treating influenza in children (Cochrane Review). In: *The Cochrane Library. Review CD002744.* Update Software, Oxford.

Monto A, Grevenstein AS, Ellitt M *et al.* (2000) Clinical signs and symptoms predict influenza infection. *Arch Int Med.* **160:** 3242–7.

Public Health Agency of Canada (2005) National Advisory Committee on Immunization (NACI). *Update of Influenza Vaccination for the 2005–2006 Season.* www.phac-aspc.gc.ca/publicat/ccdr-rmtc.

Public Health Agency of Canada (2004) *Canadian Pandemic Influenza Plan;* www.phac-aspc.gc.ca/cpic-pclcpil.

Sarnoff R and Rundell T (1999) Meta-analysis of interventions to increase influenza vaccination rates among high-risk populations. *Med Care Research and Review.* **55:** 432–56.

Shekel JJ (1992) Amantidine blocks the channel. *Nature*. **358**: 110–11.

Smits AJ, Hak E, Stalman WA *et al.* (2002) Clinical effectiveness of conventional influenza vaccination in asthmatic children. *Epidemiol Infect*. **128**: 205–11.

Soo W (1989) Adverse effects of rimantidine: summary from clinical trials. *J Resp Dis*. **10** (Suppl.): 26–31.

Stott DJ, Roberts MA and Stott D (1997) Influenza vaccination of health care works in long term care hospitals reduces the mortality of the elderly patients. *J Infect Dis*. **175**: 1–6.

Strassburg MA, Greenland S, Sorvillo FJ *et al.* (1986) Influenza in the elderly: report of an outbreak and review of vaccine effectiveness reports. *Vaccine*. **4**: 38–44.

Takahashi H, Tanala Y, Ohyama T *et al.* (2001) Evaluation of a mass influenza campaign. *Japan J Infect Dis*. **54**: 184–8.

Tan A, Bhalla P and Smyth R (2002) Vaccines for preventing influenza in people with cystic fibrosis (Cochrane Review). In: *The Cochrane Library. Review CD001753*. Update Software, Oxford.

Wilde JA, McMillan J, Serwint J *et al.* (1999) Effectiveness of influenza vaccination in health care professionals: a randomised trial. *JAMA*. **281**: 908–13.

van Elden L, van Essen GA, Boucher CA, *et al.* (2001) Clinical diagnosis of influenza virus infection: evaluation of diagnostic tools in general practice. *Br J Gen Practice*. **51**: 630–4.

van Essen GA, Kuyvenhovven MM and de Melker RA (1997) Why do healthy elderly people fail to comply with influenza vaccination? *Age Aging*. **26**: 275–9.

Chapter 9

Croup

Epidemiology and aetiology

- Croup occurs in 2–6% of children each year.
- It is most common in children under 6 years of age.
- Boys are more commonly affected than girls.
- Most cases occur in late autumn and winter.
- Most cases are mild. Only 2–4% of cases are hospitalised and only 1 in 4500 need to be intubated.

Croup occurs annually in about 6% of children during their first 5 years of life. It accounts for about 2–3% of all hospital admissions for children (Denny et al., 1983; Hendrickson et al., 1997). A study in Belgium (Van Bever, 1999) found that 16% of children had suffered from croup, and 5% of children suffered from recurrent croup (i.e. they had three or more episodes). The condition is more common in atopic children. Most children with croup have only mild symptoms. Only about 4% need to be hospitalised, and only one in 170 hospitalised children (one in 4500 of all children with croup) needs to be intubated (Chapman, 1981; Marx et al., 1997).

Although croup is a self-limiting illness, it is a large burden on healthcare systems because of the frequent visits made to doctors and emergency departments. Dr Keith Hodgkin (Hodgkin, 1978) found that croup occurred in about 1 in 50 patients per year in his English general practice, mostly in their first 5 years of life. It occurred mainly between October and April, and 30% of children reported more than one attack over a 3-year period. Croup is the cause of 250 000 emergency-room visits in the USA each year. In that country, there are biennial epidemics of croup, during the autumn months of odd-numbered years. The National Hospital Discharge Survey (Kozak et al., 2005) showed mean annual numbers of hospitalisations for croup of about 40 000, and 91% of hospitalisations occurred in children under 5 years of age.

There is a higher incidence of croup in Caucasian children – about threefold higher – than in African-American children. Boys get croup more often than girls, and a systematic review (Phelan *et al.*, 1982) found that 72% of sufferers in croup trials were male.

Families with a history of asthma were more likely to have children who suffered from croup, presumably due to the presence of hyper-reactive airways. The annual incidence in children under 6 years of age ranged from 1.5% to 6%. The hospital admission rates for children with croup ranged from 1.5% to 31% of cases seen. These wide variations reflect differences in hospital admission practices and the severity of the condition in the population being assessed (Marx *et al.*, 1997)

Although most children suffer only mildly with the illness for a short period, croup causes anxiety for parents and GPs, and 2–4% of children with croup are admitted to hospital. However, only about 2% of those admitted to hospital require intubation to help their breathing, and the mortality rate is now very low.

- The cause of croup is usually viral.
- Parainfluenza virus types 1 and 3 are the most common, but influenza A and B viruses, adenovirus and respiratory syncytial virus have also been implicated.
- *Mycoplasma pneumoniae* is occasionally implicated.

Croup is almost always a viral infection. Parainfluenza types 1 and 3 are the commonest causative agents (Denny, 1983). Influenza virus types A and B, adenoviruses and respiratory syncytial viruses have also been isolated (Chapman, 1981). *Mycoplasma pneumoniae* has occasionally been implicated, and enterovirus, mumps virus, measles virus, rhinovirus and *Corynebacterium diphtheriae* have rarely been isolated. Thus the same viruses that cause the common cold, influenza, bronchitis and sinusitis in other children and adults also cause croup.

Clinical course and treatment

The specific symptoms of croup are usually preceded by those of a non-specific ARI, such as cough, rhinorrhoea and fever. Viral invasion of the child's laryngeal mucosa leads to inflammation, hyperaemia, epithelial necrosis and shedding of cells from this region. This leads to narrowing and irritation of the subglottic region, which causes the child to breathe more quickly and deeply. Airflow through the upper airway becomes more turbulent. In moderate cases the pliant chest wall caves in during inspiration, and in severe cases the child becomes fatigued, hypoxic and hypercapnoeic. The characteristic barking seal-like cough, inspiratory stridor and respiratory distress usually develop fairly quickly during the evening or night. Inspiratory stridor is typical, and fever can occur (up to 40°C). The symptoms are usually worse at night, and improve during the day.

The majority of children with croup are only mildly ill, and their symptoms resolve within 48 hours, although a small percentage of children can have symptoms that last for 5 to 6 days. When a child's condition deteriorates, it does so at a rate that usually enables healthcare professionals to take action. Children with croup are often categorised as having mild, moderate, severe or impending respiratory failure. Although it is clear that the latter two categories require urgent inpatient treatment, there is debate about the extent to which the first two categories can be safely managed in general practice.

How is the doctor to assess the severity of illness, and the likelihood of inpatient treatment, in an individual child? Various croup scores have been developed, but the existence of several scores sometimes makes comparison of study results difficult. The earliest and still the most commonly used scale was developed by Westley (Westley, 1978) and is a 17-point scale. One of the problems with these ordinal scales is that they were developed before pulse oximetry became widely available, and they therefore do not take oximetry readings into account. Most doctors rely on their clinical judgement when assessing the severity of croup.

- Supportive care for croup patients:
  - explain the illness to the parents
  - keep the child and their parents together
  - give an analgesic/antipyretic.
- There is no evidence for the efficacy of humidified air.
- Nebulised epinephrine is rapidly effective in improving symptoms.
- Oral, nebulised or intramuscular dexamethasone is effective in relieving symptoms at 6 hours and 12 hours, but there is no additional effect at 24 hours.
- Steroids:
  - reduce symptoms
  - reduce the number of hospitalisations
  - reduce intubations
  - reduce time in hospital
  - reduce the duration of illness
  - reduce the number of subsequent healthcare visits.
- A single dose of steroid is usually effective.

There is a large and increasing amount of literature on the inpatient management of the more severe cases of croup in hospital or paediatric emergency centers, and there are studies and reviews that provide good evidence for effective management of such cases (Fitzgerald and Kilhan, 2003; Alberta Medical Association, 2004). Unfortunately, there is very little evidence concerning the optimum management of the milder cases of croup that constitute the majority, and are usually treated by GPs.

If a small child has a barky cough and stridor, croup is almost invariably present, and most doctors have no difficulty in making the diagnosis. Although bacterial tracheitis and acute epiglottitis are rare, it is important to exclude them. Children with these conditions tend to have a higher fever, without preceding common cold symptoms. Often tracheitis is not diagnosed until a child has proved unresponsive to the standard croup medications. The child with epiglottitis will appear toxic, will be drooling and will not have the typical cough of croup. Since the development of the HIB vaccine, such children are much more rarely seen.

It is difficult to advise GPs how to manage croup, even though they manage the vast majority of children with the condition. There have been no randomised controlled trials or systematic reviews evaluating interventions versus placebo in true primary care settings. The bulk of the literature discusses how to manage the more serious minority of cases who attend Emergency Departments and are admitted to hospital.

Supportive care

The relatively sudden and nocturnal nature of croup symptoms is very alarming for parents, and commonly results in a visit to an Emergency Department. It is important to educate the parents about the self-limited nature of the disease, and to advise them on how to recognise when the child's condition is getting worse.

It is traditional to treat children with croup with humidified air. In the nineteenth and early twentieth centuries, special 'croup kettles' were marketed to give this treatment. Unfortunately, despite the long history of kettle use, there is no good evidence that humidified air is an effective intervention. A randomised trial by Dr Gina Neto and colleagues at the University of Ottawa (Neto, 2002) studied 70 Canadian children with moderate croup, all of whom were treated in the Emergency Department with oral dexamethasone, and half of whom received humidified oxygen through a mist stick. Both groups improved, but there was no difference with regard to improvement of croup scores between the group that received humidified oxygen through a mist stick and the group that did not. A critical review (Levine and Scolnik, 2001) found no evidence of benefit from mist; and one well-designed moderate-sized study and two small studies have failed to show a benefit. Mist is no longer advised, especially the use of mist tents, which separate the child from the parents.

Most general practitioners can provide anecdotal evidence that children often seem to improve on their way to the clinic or Emergency Department in the middle of a cold winter night. It makes physiological sense that inflamed tissues may shrink on contact with cold air. However, there is no evidence in the literature to support this intervention.

Pharmacotherapy

Antipyretics/antitussives and decongestants

There is no evidence from controlled trials to indicate whether children with feverish croup should be given antipyretics. However, most authorities consider it reasonable to offer them as a comfort measure. No experimental studies have been published regarding any potential benefit of antitussives and anticongestants for children with croup. They should probably not be given, although most parents will have administered them by the time the doctor sees the patient.

Oxygen/helium

If the child is hypoxic, oxygen should be given. It would seem natural to give oxygen to all children with croup. However, its use is now recommended only for children with an oxygen saturation of 92% or less in room air. A few years ago, administration of helium to children with croup was advocated because of its potential (because of the lower density of the gas) to decrease the turbulence of airflow through the narrowed airway. However, several studies have failed to show any clear evidence that it has such a benefit (McGee *et al.*, 1997).

Antibiotics

As croup is a viral illness, there is no point in giving antibiotics. However, it is not uncommon to see a child with croup who has been given an antibiotic for a preceding common cold or cough.

Systemic corticosteroids

Many individual studies in different parts of the world have found administration of steroids to children with croup to be beneficial. For example, in a trial in Cleveland conducted by Dr Dennis Super and colleagues (Super *et al.*, 1990), children hospitalised with croup were given either intramuscular dexamethasone or a saline placebo. Twelve hours after the injection, the dexamethasone-treated patients showed a significant decline in median croup score from 4.5 to 1.0. By 24 hours a decrease of 2 points or more in the croup score was found in 85% of the dexamethasone group and only 33% of the placebo group. During this period, only 19% of dexamethasone-treated patients needed two or more racemic epinephrine treatments, compared with 62% of the placebo group. Similarly, in Detroit a trial (Cruz *et al.*, 1995) of a single intramuscular injection of dexamethasone administered to children aged from 6 months to 5 years attending an Emergency Department found that 21% of the placebo group sought follow-up care, compared with 5% in the treatment group. After 24 hours, 84% of the treatment group reported an improvement in symptoms, compared with 42% of the control group.

There have now been at least 24 published randomised trials of the use of steroids to treat croup (most of these trials have been done in paediatric emergency departments or in-patient wards, not in general practice). A review for the Cochrane Collaboration by Ausejo *et al.* (Ausejo *et al.*, 2002; Kairys *et al.*, 1989) found that glucocorticoid treatment was associated with an improvement in the croup severity score at 6 hours (NNT = 7) and 12 hours (NNT = 5), but after 24 hours there was no significant difference between the intervention and control groups. There was a decrease in adrenaline given, a decrease in the length of time spent in the Emergency Department, and a decrease in the number of hospital admissions. For inpatients, the mean reduction in duration of hospital stay was 16 hours. Not only were the symptoms of croup significantly improved, but also the number of subsequent admissions to hospital was reduced (NNT *c.*2). In addition, in the week following administration of the steroid, there were lower rates of re-attendance to any doctor or hospital (number needed to prevent one additional child re-attending = *c.*12). Another review, by Kairys *et al.* (1989), found that children who are given systemic steroids when they are admitted to hospital with croup have significantly improved symptom scores after 12 hours (NNT *c.*7) as well as reduced duration of hospital stay. Steroids have been shown to reduce the number and duration of intubations and to reduce the rate of re-intubations. The reviews suggested that steroids might be slightly less effective when given by nebuliser than when administered by injection or by mouth. It was concluded that 'The degree of benefit of a number needed to treat of 5 to 7 is sufficient to justify the use of glucocorticoids in all patients with croup' (Kairys, 1989).

A group in Cardiff headed by Dr Robin Parker studied 188 children with croup who had been treated with oral prednisone, to see how long stridor at rest persisted after steroid treatment. The median duration of persistent stridor was 6.5 hours. It was concluded that 'Stridor at rest resolves promptly after the administration of oral steroids in the vast majority of cases. This suggests that many patients previously treated in hospital may be able to be treated and discharged from the ED' (Parker *et al.*, 2004)

All the trial evidence discussed so far is for children with moderate to severe croup, treated as inpatients, usually with intramuscular steroids. In a recently completed large multi-centre trial in Canada, conducted by Dr Candice Bjornson and colleagues (Bjornson *et al.*, 2004), and involving 720 children with mild croup (defined as a score of 2 or less on the Westley scale), it was found that children who had been treated with oral dexamethasone returned half as often to a healthcare centre compared with children in the placebo group (7% vs. 15%). They also had substantially less severe croup symptoms, and less lost sleep in the 48 hours following treatment. Their parents experienced less stress in the 24 hours following treatment, and the costs to both the families and the healthcare system were slightly lower. The benefit appeared to be just as great in children with very mild symptoms (only a barky cough) as in those who had had croup symptoms for several days at the time of treatment. It was concluded that 'For children with mild croup, dexamethasone is an effective treatment that results in consistent and small but important clinical and economic benefits. Although the long-term effects of this treatment are not known, our data support the use of dexamethasone in most, if not all, children with croup' (Bjornson *et al.*, 2004).

Dexamethasone appears to be equally effective whether given orally or parenterally. A trial in the USA involving 126 children with moderate to severe croup (Donaldson, 2003), which compared the two routes of administration in an Emergency Department, found that at 24 hours and 10 days after treatment with either oral or intramuscular steroid, there were no statistically significant differences between the two groups with regard to the presence of stridor, expiratory sounds, barky cough and sleep disturbance, the degree of improvement, or the proportion in whom there was complete resolution of symptoms after one day. Most doctors prefer to give oral treatment, as this is less painful for the child. Most children with croup will not vomit the medication.

No controlled studies have been published that examine whether or not multiple doses of corticosteroids are of greater benefit than a single dose. Given that untreated croup is typically a disease of short duration, a single dose of corticosteroid is probably sufficient for most patients.

Inhaled steroids

The same reviews have shown that steroids given by nebuliser rather than by injection are also effective. This treatment halved both the likelihood of a poor outcome and the rate of hospital admission (NNT *c*.4) (Kairys, 1989; Ausejo, 2002). For example, in a Danish study of children who were admitted to hospital with moderate to severe croup, and randomised to either inhaled budesonide or saline inhalation; two hours after treatment there was a significant decrease in the croup symptom score in the treatment group (Mortensen *et al.*, 1994). Inhaled budenoside is more difficult to administer than an injection, and it is more expensive. Its only likely use is in a severely ill child who cannot take medicine by mouth. A systematic review by Griffin *et al.* (2000) assessed the effectiveness of treatment with nebulised steroids for children with croup. They found eight good-quality randomised trials. Children who had been treated with nebulised steroids were more likely to show an improvement in croup scores after 5 hours, and were less likely to require hospital admission after attending an Emergency Department.

Some physicians feel that there is a need for further trials to define the indications for and effectiveness of steroid treatment of mild croup in the community. Others feel that in view of the comparative safety and low cost of dexamethasone, it makes sense to continue using glucocorticoids for all children with croup. Oral dexamethasone should be the treatment of choice, because of its safety and efficacy. In a child who is vomiting, nebulised or intramuscular injection might be preferable.

Nebulised adrenaline (epinephrine)

Epinephrine has been shown to substantially reduce respiratory distress within 10 minutes, and to be effective for more than 1 hour. However, all of its effects wear off within 2 hours. There have been no systematic reviews of the use of epinephrine, although it has been extensively used since the 1960s, when Westley and colleagues (Westley *et al.*, 1978) conducted a randomised trial on only 20 children! They found that the clinical scores in the treatment group were significantly improved after 10 and 30 minutes, but not after 120 minutes. Similar small trials in Sweden and Washington have found that nebulised adrenaline caused a reduction in croup symptom scores compared with placebo (Waisman *et al.*, 1992; Kristjannson, 1994). The Washington trial, conducted by Dr Yehezkel Waisman and colleagues, also found that racemic and 1:1000 L-epinephrine are equally effective as aerosols (Waisman *et al.*, 1992). The same dose of either preparation is used in children of all ages and sizes. The relative size of the child's tidal volume is thought to modulate the amount of drug that is actually delivered to the child's upper airway.

Adrenaline (epinephrine) plus steroids

Two cohort studies (Ledwith *et al.*, 1995; Kunkel and Baker, 1996) have looked at the effects of using adrenaline combined with steroids, given in a paediatric assessment unit. It was found that 60% of children were discharged within 4 hours. A study in an Emergency Department in

Grand Falls, Michigan (Prendergast *et al.*, 1994), attempted to identify a cohort of children with croup who may be safely discharged after treatment with racemic epinephrine, corticosteroids and observation. If a child had persistent resting stridor or a croup score greater than 2 on the Westley scale 60 minutes after the start of therapy, hospitalisation was required. Otherwise, children could go home. None of these children re-attended for further medical care during the following 2 days. A number of retrospective and prospective studies (not trials) suggest that patients who are treated with epinephrine may be safely discharged home so long as their symptoms have not recurred 2 or 3 hours after treatment.

Most centres now use both epinephrine and corticosteroids to treat children with croup. The epinephrine acts quickly to produce relief until the slower-acting steroid begins to work, and the steroid action persists long after the epinephrine effect has worn off.

References

Alberta Medical Association (2004) *Guidelines for the Diagnosis and Management of Croup*. www.albertadoctors.org

Ausejo M, Saentz A and Pham B (2002) Glucocorticoids for croup (Cochrane Review). In: *The Cochrane Library. Review CD001955*. Update Software, Oxford.

Bjornson C, Klassen TP, Williamson J and Brant R (2004) A randomized trial of a single dose of oral dexamethasone for mild croup. *NEJM*. **351**: 306–13.

Chapman R (1981) The epidemiology of tracheobronchitis in paediatric practice. *Am J Epidemiol*. **114**: 786–97.

Cruz MN, Stewart G and Rosenberg N (1995) Use of dexamethasone in the outpatient management of acute laryngo-tracheitis. *Paediatrics*. **96**: 220–3.

Denny FW, Murphy TF, Cldye WA, Collier AM and Henderson FW (1983) An 11-year study of croup in a pediatric practice. *Pediatrics*. **71**: 871–6.

Donaldson D (2003) Intramuscular versus oral dexamethasone for moderate to severe croup: a randomized double-blind trial. *Academic Emergency Medicine*. **10**: 16–21.

Fitzgerald DA and Kilham HA (2003) Croup: Assessment and evidence-based management. *Med J Aust*. **179**: 372–7.

Griffin S, Ellis S, Fitzgerald-Barron A, Rose J and Egger M (2000) Nebulised steroid in the treatment of croup: a systematic review of randomized controlled trials. *Br J Gen Pract*. **50**: 135–41.

Henrickson KJ, Kuhn SM and Savatski LL (1997) Epidemiology and cost of infections with human parainfluenza virus types 1 and 2 in young children. *Clin Infect Dis*. **18**: 770–9.

Hodgkin K (1978) *Towards Earlier Diagnosis in Primary Care* (4e) Churchill Livingstone, New York.

Kairys SW, Olmstead EM and O'Connor GT (1989) Steroid treatment of laryngo-tracheitis: a meta-analysis of the evidence from randomized trials. *Paediatrics*. **83**: 683–93.

Kozak LJ, Owings MF and Hall MJ (2005) National Hospital Discharge Survey, 2002. Annual summary with detailed diagnosis and procedure data. *Vital Health Stat*. **158**: 1–199.

Kristjannson S, Berg-Kelly K and Winso E (1994) Inhalation of racemic adrenaline in the treatment of mild or moderately severe croup. *Acta Paediatr.* **83**: 1156–60.

Kunkel NC and Baker MD (1996) Use of racemic epinephrine, dexamethasone and mist in the outpatient management of croup. *Paed Emerg Care.* **12**: 156–9.

Ledwith CA, Shea LM and Mauro RA (1995) Safety and efficacy of nebulized epinephrine in conjunction with oral dexamethasone and mist in the outpatient treatment of croup. *Annals Emerg Med.* **25**: 331–7.

Levine E and Scolnik D (2001) Lack of efficacy of humidification in the treatment of croup: why do physicians persist in using an unproven modality? *Can J Emerg Med.* **1**: 209–12.

Marx A, Torok TJ, Holman RC *et al.* (1997) Pediatric hospitalization for croup – biennial increases with human parainfluenza virus 1 epidemics. *J Infect Dis.* **176**: 1423–7.

McGee DL, Wald DA and Hinchcliffe S (1997) Helium/oxygen therapy in the emergency department. *J Emerg Med.* **15**: 291–6.

Mortensen S, Agertoft L, Husby S and Pederson S (1994) Pseudo-croup treated with inhaled steroid. A double-blind placebo-controlled trial. *Ugeskr Laeger.* **156**: 6661–3.

Neto GM (2002) A randomized controlled trial of mist in the acute treatment of moderate croup. *Acad Emerg Medicine.* **9**: 873–89.

Parker R, Powell CV and Kelly AM (2004) How long does stridor at rest persist in croup after the administration of oral prednisolone? *Emerg Med Aust.* **16**: 135–8.

Phelan PD, Landau LI and Olinsily A (1982) *Respiratory Illness in Children* (2e) Blackwell Science, Oxford.

Prendergast M, Jones JS and Hartman D (1994) Racemic epinephrine in the treatment of croup – can we identify children for outpatient therapy? *Am J Emerg Med.* **12**: 613–16.

Super DM, Cartelli NA, Brooks LJ *et al.* (1990) A prospective randomized double-blind study to evaluate the effect of dexamethasone in acute tracheobronchitis. *J Pediatr.* **116**: 667–8.

van Bever HP, Wieringa MH and Weyler JJ (1999) Current and recurrent croup; their association with asthma and allergy. *Eur J Paed.* **158**: 253–57.

Waisman Y, Klein BL, Boenning DA, Young GM and Chamberlain JM (1992) Prospective randomized double-blind study comparing ʟ-epinephrine and racemic epinephrine aerosols in the treatment of croup. *Pediatrics.* **89**: 302–6.

Westley CR, Cotton EK and Brooks JG (1978) Nebulized racemic epinephrine by IPPB for the treatment of croup: a double-blind study. *Am J Dis Child.* **132**: 44–7.

Chapter 10

Bronchiolitis

Epidemiology and aetiology

- Bronchiolitis is the commonest lower respiratory tract infection in infants.
- Around 1–2% of children under 12 months of age are hospitalised each year. Only 1% of hospitalised children die of the illness.
- The mean duration of hospital stay is 3–4 days.
- Bronchiolitis occurs mainly in winter.
- The incidence of bronchiolitis is increasing.
- Around 80–100% of cases are due to the respiratory syncytial virus (RSV).

Bronchiolitis is the commonest lower respiratory tract infection in infants. Almost all children will have experienced one lower respiratory infection by 24 months of age, and half of them will have had two or more infections (Phelan *et al.*, 1994). Like croup, it occurs in a seasonal pattern, with the highest incidence in winter. In warmer climates, its incidence peaks during the rainy season. Each year in the USA around 20% of infants are said to have lower respiratory tract infections, but only 1–2% of children under 12 months of age are admitted to hospital each year (Gruber *et al.*, 1997).

Bronchiolitis is the leading cause of hospitalisation of infants younger than 1 year, and over 80% of children hospitalised are under 6 months of age. The peak rate of admission occurs in infants aged 2–6 months. The illness is more common in premature infants and in children under 6 weeks old, and in infants with congenital heart disease and children with chronic lung disease. Disease severity is directly related to the size and maturity of the infant. Other factors associated with a prolonged or complicated history include a history of apnoea or respiratory arrest, pulmonary consolidation and Native American or Inuit ethnic origin (Glezen *et al.*, 1981). In the Netherlands, the rate of hospitalisations due to bronchiolitis increased between 1991 and 1999, whereas the rates due to asthma and pneumonia did not (van Woensel and van Aalderan 2002).

Similarly, in Canada, between 1980 and 2000 the rate of hospitalisation for bronchiolitis increased in all provinces, especially in children under 6 months of age (Langley *et al.*, 2003; Wang *et al.*, 1995). On the other hand, mean length of stay in hospital decreased from 5.4 to 3.1 days. A concurrent increase in other respiratory diagnostic codes was not seen in either country, so this trend over two decades may indicate a change in either the prevalence or severity of bronchiolitis.

The risk of death for a healthy infant with respiratory syncytial virus (RSV) bronchiolitis is less than 0.5%, but the risk of death within 2 weeks is much higher for children with congenital heart disease (3.5%) and chronic lung disease (3.45%). High-risk children have a 35% chance of being admitted to an intensive-care unit, and 20% of them require mechanical ventilation (Navas *et al.*, 1992).

Does bronchiolitis cause, or is it associated with, subsequent asthma? The evidence is conflicting. Two small prospective studies (McConnaichie *et al.*, 1985; Sly and Hibbert 1989) found that children who had suffered from bronchiolitis were not at increased risk of developing asthma. Another follow-up study (McConnaichie and Roughmann, 1986) of 50 infants who had been admitted with bronchiolitis found that 5 years later their asthma incidence rate was double that of the general population.

RSV is responsible for 70% of bronchiolitis, and this figure rises to 80–100% in winter epidemics. However, in the early spring the parainfluenza virus type 3 is often responsible, as it is for croup. The annual cost of RSV-associated illness was almost $18 million in Canada in 1993 (Wang, 1995), and 10 times that in the USA (Gruber, 1997).

- The diagnosis of bronchiolitis is based on clinical findings, namely wheezing in the presence of respiratory infection symptoms. Tests are of little value.
- The mean duration of illness is 10 days, but some children are sick for up to 1 month.
- Hospitalisation should be considered if:
  - the infant is premature
  - the infant is less than 3 months old
  - the respiratory rate is more than 70 breaths per minute
  - oxygen saturation is less than 92% in room air
  - the infant has cardiopulmonary disease
  - the infant is immunodeficient
  - the infant is lethargic.

Bronchiolitis is a virally induced bronchiolar inflammation that is associated with signs and symptoms of airway obstruction. Diagnosis is based on clinical findings, namely fever, rhinitis, tachypnoea, expiratory wheezing, flaring of the nostrils, and intercostal chest wall retractions. Until it has been proved otherwise, a wheezing infant is assumed to have bronchiolitis. The illness has a mean duration of about 10 days in infants, but 10% of infants remain unwell after 4 weeks. Bronchiolitis is sometimes classified clinically as mild (not requiring hospitalisation), moderate (requiring hospitalisation but not intubation) or severe (requiring intubation or artificial ventilation). Unfortunately, there is no reliable and validated clinical score for bronchiolitis, which means that these terms are used differently by different authors.

Most children with RSV infection, who have only a mild illness, can be treated at home so long as they are closely supervised by parents or caregivers who have been warned what to look for. Signs that the condition is worsening include an increasing respiratory rate, onset of laboured breathing (use of accessory muscles, retractions, cyanosis or flared nostrils), fewer wet nappies, temperature greater than 38°C, or an overall worsening appearance (American Academy of Pediatrics, 2003).

The American Academy of Pediatrics (2003) recommends that the following categories of children should be hospitalised when they contract bronchiolitis: age less than 3 months; gestational age at birth less than 34 weeks; children with cardiopulmonary disease; children with immunodeficiencies; respiratory rate more than 70 breaths/minute; lethargic appearance; wheezing and respiratory distress associated with an oxygen saturation of less than 92% in room air; hypercarbia; atelectasis or consolidation on chest X-ray.

The diagnosis of bronchiolitis is based on the history and the results of an examination. As mentioned above, until it has been proved otherwise, all wheezing infants are assumed to have bronchiolitis. A review by Dr Clayton Bordley of Duke University Medical Center in North Carolina (Bordley *et al.*, 2004) found that although the rapid RSV antigen tests have acceptable sensitivity and specificity, there is no evidence that performing this test affects the clinical outcomes in typical cases. Although chest X-rays are usually taken, the number that showed abnormality has been found to range from 20% to 90% in different studies (Bordley *et al.* 2004), and there are insufficient data to demonstrate that chest X-ray films reliably distinguish between viral and bacterial infections. Furthermore, blood counts do not correlate with chest X-ray results. The authors of the review concluded that 'The many studies to date do not define clear value for any test; given the high prevalence of the disease, prospective studies of the utility of the various testing modalities are needed'.

In Canada, the Pediatric Investigators Collaborative Network on Infections in Canada (which delights in its jolly acronym, PICNIC) has conducted several good-quality studies of bronchiolitis. It studied inter-observer variation in clinical assessment of bronchiolitis, in eight paediatric centres, with regard to history of apnoea, assessment of cyanosis, respiratory rate, chest retractions, oximetry and reason for hospitalization (Wang *et al.*, 1996). There was strong agreement on a history of apnoea and assessment of cyanosis, but there was wide variation in agreement about other features. The authors suggested that there was a need for more standardised training, to ensure consistent and reproducible assessment. Another study, by Dr Dmitri Christakis of the University of Washington (Christakis *et al.*, 2005) looked at inpatient diagnostic testing and management of bronchiolitis in 30 large children's hospitals in the USA. The mean length of stay in hospital ranged from 2.4 to 3.9 days, and there was wide variation in the use of diagnostic tests and medications, as well as in re-admission rates. The factors associated with increased length of stay were higher severity scores and the use of antibiotics, bronchodilators and corticosteroids.

Treatment of bronchiolitis

- There is no one effective treatment for bronchiolitis.
- Treatments that may possibly be effective include the following:
  - nebulised epinephrine
  - beta-agonists
  - ipratropium
  - corticosteroids
  - oxygen.
- Treatments that are of little value include the following:
  - ribavirin
  - antibiotics
  - nursing measures.
- Treatments that are of possible value for prophylaxis in premature and high-risk infants include the following:
  - monoclonal antibody
  - RSV immunoglobulin.
- As yet there is no effective RSV vaccine.

Common-sense measures for care are usually advised. Home-made salt-water drops can help to mobilise nasal mucus (the drops should be applied before suctioning). Hands should be washed and visiting limited in order to prevent transmission. Exposure to tobacco smoke should be avoided. However, there is only limited evidence that these common-sense measures help to control the spread of infection.

Physicians have tried many different drugs, and combinations of drugs, to help infants with bronchiolitis. The presence of so many agents almost suggests a sense of desperation. A technical report published by the Agency for Healthcare Research and Quality (2003) in the USA reviewed the evidence concerning agents for the treatment and prevention of bronchiolitis. It found that the evidence base was limited, as many trials were small, with insufficient statistical power to permit an accurate assessment of the efficacy of the therapeutic agents being investigated. It is possible that some of the agents are effective for bronchiolitis, and that we just don't have the evidence for them yet. A very balanced review of the treatment options for acute bronchiolitis has recently been published by Dr Robert Steiner of the University of Louisville School of Medicine. He concluded that at best it is only possible to label some interventions 'possibly effective' (Steiner, 2004).

The PICNIC group studied the admission and management of 1516 patients treated at nine different hospitals in Canada. Significant differences were observed in the proportion of patients with underlying disease, aged less than 6 weeks, with hypoxia, and whether pulmonary infiltrate was detected on chest X-ray. The mean length of stay in hospital ranged from 8.6 to 11.8 days, and there was variation between hospitals in the interventions used, in both compromised and previously healthy patients. It was concluded that 'Variation exists in pediatric hospitals in the nature of patients admitted with RSV bronchiolitis; there is also widespread variation in the interventions used by hospitals' (Wang *et al.*, 1996).

The situation with regard to pharmacological treatment of bronchiolitis is well summed up by a recent systematic review (King *et al.*, 2004) by researchers at the University of North Carolina: 'Overall, little evidence supports a routine role for any drug in treating patients with bronchiolitis. A sufficiently large, well-designed pragmatic trial of the commonly used interventions for bronchiolitis (epinephrine, beta-2-agonists, corticosteroids, anticholinergics) is needed to determine the most effective treatment strategies for managing this condition.' Another review, by Dr Job van Woensel of the Emma Children's Hospital in Amsterdam (van Woensel and Kimpen, 2000) found that 'Attempts to find an effective therapy have so far been unsuccessful. Symptomatic therapy with bronchodilators may give only short-term relief of symptoms in some patients; the effect of corticosteroids and ribavirin has been disappointing.'

Thus there is a clear lack of evidence for any effective interventions that will help infants with acute bronchiolitis. Nevertheless, there are suggestions that some therapies may be useful. Let us examine the contenders.

Bronchodilators

Individual randomised trials initially presented an optimistic picture of the use of bronchodilators. For example, Dr Terry Klassen and her colleagues at the University of Ottawa (Klassen *et al.*, 1991) compared nebulised salbutamol with saline as control in children of median age 6 months with bronchiolitis. Patients in the salbutamol group showed significantly greater improvement in clinical scores, but no difference in oxygen saturation. The findings of later studies were not so positive. One systematic review, by Kellner *et al.* (2001), evaluated children who had been treated with bronchodilators in Emergency Departments and after admission to hospital. In total, eight randomised controlled trials were found. In the short term, bronchodilators lowered clinical scores in children with mild or moderate bronchiolitis. The authors concluded that 'Bronchodilators produce a modest short-term improvement in clinical scores; this small benefit must be weighed against the costs of these agents.' Dr Glenn Flores of Boston University School of Medicine attempted to perform a meta-analysis on studies of the efficacy of beta-2-agonists used in outpatient settings only. The trials were so variable that no satisfactory analysis could be done. He found that beta-2-agonists had no impact on either hospitalisation or respiratory rate, but had a statistically significant but clinically non-significant effect on oxygen saturation level and heart rate. He summarised the situation by stating that 'Conclusive evidence for the efficacy of beta-2-agonist therapy for bronchiolitis remains unavailable' (Flores and Horwitz, 1997). There was no evidence in either review that the use of bronchodilators decreased the rate of hospital admission from outpatient or Emergency Department settings. The reviewers found that the evidence for the effectiveness of bronchodilators was weak: 'Bronchodilators may transiently improve the clinical appearance of the child through a general stimulatory effect, rather than by improving respiratory function' (Flores and Horwitz, 1997).

Another Cochrane Review, by Lisa Hartling and colleagues at the University of Alberta, examined the evidence for the effectiveness of epinephrine in the treatment of bronchiolitis (Hartling *et al*, 2001). A total of 14 studies were found. Among the inpatient trials that compared epinephrine with placebo, there was only one significant outcome that favoured epinephrine (an improvement in clinical score after 60 minutes). For outpatient trials, change in clinical score after 60 minutes, change in oxygen saturation after 30 minutes, respiratory rate after 30 minutes and 'overall clinical improvement' favoured epinephrine. Admission rates were not significantly different. The reviewers concluded that 'There is some evidence to suggest that epinephrine may be better than placebo in outpatients; there is insufficient evidence to support the use of epinephrine for the treatment of bronchiolitis among inpatients' (Hartling *et al.*, 2001).

Anticholinergic medications

A Cochrane Review by Dr Mark Everard and colleagues at Sheffield University found six trials. Anticholinergic medications are often used, but their efficacy is uncertain. Compared with a beta-2-agonist alone, the combination of ipratropium and a beta-2-agonist was associated with a reduced need for additional treatment, but no difference was found in treatment response, respiratory rate or oxygen saturation improvement in the Emergency Department. There was no significant difference in length of hospital stay when ipratropium alone was compared with placebo. However, the combination of ipratropium and a beta-2-agonist resulted in a significantly improved clinical score after 24 hours, compared with placebo. The authors concluded that 'There is not enough evidence to support the uncritical use of anticholinergic therapy for wheezing infants, although parents using it at home were able to identify improvements' (Everard *et al.*, 2001).

Corticosteroids

Ever since it became apparent that corticosteroids are an effective intervention for children with croup, it has been hoped that they would be equally efficacious in bronchiolitis. Unfortunately, the evidence for a beneficial effect is not strong.

A meta-analysis by Dr Michelle Garrison and colleagues at the University of Washington found that infants who received steroids had a mean length of hospital stay just under half a day less than those who did not, half a day less of symptoms, and a lower clinical symptom score. The authors concluded that 'Steroids produce a statistically significant effect' (Garrison *et al.*, 2000). A Cochrane Review undertaken later by Dr Hema Patel and colleagues at the Montreal Children's Hospital (and which included several more recent studies than the first review) found that there was no significant decrease in length of stay in hospital, no difference in clinical scores, no differences in hospital admission rates and re-admission rates, and no difference in oxygen saturation levels or respiratory rate. The authors concluded that 'The available evidence suggests that corticosteroid therapy is of no benefit in this patient group' (Patel *et al.*, 2000). The discrepancies in the results of the two reviews can be partly explained by the difficulty that the reviewers had in coping with the different scales and methods used to measure the clinical state of the children. The results were often too heterogeneous to allow useful comparisons to be made, and some studies included children with a previous diagnosis of asthma. It was concluded that 'Even if there is an effect, its size is likely to be very small, and has to be weighed against the acute adverse effects of corticosteroids' (Patel *et al.*, 2000).

Post-bronchiolitis wheezing has been described in several studies. It was hoped that the use of corticosteroids during the acute phase of bronchiolitis might reduce subsequent wheezing. Unfortunately, this has not proved to be the case. Studies in the Netherlands (van Woensel et al., 2000) and Finland (Reijonen et al., 2000) both found that there was no difference in subsequent wheezing between children treated with steroids and those given placebo. RSV infection does not seem to be a very strong predictor of subsequent wheezing.

Bronchodilators plus steroids

Dr Laurie Goebel and colleagues at the University of South Alabama treated children who had first-time wheezing and symptoms of respiratory tract infection with albuterol plus either prednisolone or placebo for 5 days (Goebel et al., 2000). On day 2, children treated with prednisolone had significantly lower symptom scores. This difference had disappeared by day 6, which suggests that the addition of prednisolone transiently accelerates recovery from bronchiolitis. This confirmed the result of an earlier study (Tal et al., 1983), which found that the combination of dexamethasone and salbutamol resulted in a swifter resolution of bronchiolitis symptoms than either agent alone.

Antibiotics

Although doctors very often use antibiotics to treat feverish wheezing children, there appears to be only one trial which evaluated the effects of antibiotics in bronchiolitis (Friis et al., 1984) by comparing routine use of antibiotics with placebo. A total of 138 children were admitted to hospital with clinically apparent pneumonia (in 45% of cases RSV was subsequently isolated). There was no evidence that the antibiotics reduced the length of stay in hospital or that they improved clinical symptoms, clinical signs or radiographic appearance. With the increasing acceptance that bronchiolitis is almost always caused by infection of susceptible children with RSV, the consensus is that antibiotics are rarely needed.

Ribavirin and immunoglobulins

As antibiotics had proved to be ineffective, attention shifted to antiviral agents. The one used for RSV infections is ribavirin, which has only been used on small numbers of seriously ill or at-risk children in hospital. A systematic review by Randolph and Wang (2001) of 10 small trials found that, for infants and children hospitalised with bronchiolitis, administration of ribavirin compared with placebo did not reduce rates of respiratory deterioration or death. The reviewers concluded that the trials of ribavirin had insufficient power to provide reliable estimates of effects. There were some trends – the mortality rate was slightly lower when ribavirin was used (5.8% vs. 9.7%), the probability of respiratory deterioration was lower (7.1% vs. 18.3%), and there were 1.2 fewer ventilation days and 1.9 fewer days of hospitalisation.

A Cochrane Review by Wang and Tang (1999) from the Hospital for Sick Children in Toronto identified four immunoglobulin studies. Three of these studies used RSV hyperimmune globulin and one used monoclonal RSV antibody (palivizumab). These agents were given to children at high risk from underlying congenital heart disease or bronchopulmonary dysplasia. The incidence of hospitalisation (NNT = 17) and the incidence of ICU admission (NNT = 50) were halved, but the incidence of mechanical ventilation was not. Unfortunately, these trials and one subsequent trial were all small and underpowered. None of them reduced duration of hospital stay, duration of ventilation or duration of treatment with supplementary oxygen. RSV immunoglobulin can cause elevation of liver enzymes, and causes adverse effects in about 3% of children. There is currently no good evidence for the use of these agents to treat moderate or severe cases.

Despite the lack of strong evidence, the American Academy of Pediatrics (2003) currently recommends that monoclonal antibody (palivizumab) or RSV immunoglobulin should be given to the following categories of patient:

- children under 2 years of age with chronic lung disease
- preterm infants born at 28 weeks or less
- infants born at 29–32 weeks, during their first RSV season
- infants born at 32–35 weeks who are attending a childcare centre, have school-aged siblings, are exposed to environmental pollution, or have abnormalities of the airways or severe neuromuscular problems.

Palivizumab is the preferred agent for prophylaxis because it is given as five once-monthly injections, starting just before the RSV season begins in November.

Prophylaxis

If there are no effective interventions to improve the course of RSV infections that cause bronchiolitis, can the disease be prevented, especially in vulnerable children?

Although there is evidence that breastfeeding during the first 13 weeks of life protects against respiratory infective illness in the first 2 years of life, and that this is particularly true in developing countries, where breastfeeding can lower the frequency and duration of acute respiratory infection and infective diarrhoea, it is less certain whether breastfeeding is protective in developed countries. A study at the Influenza Research Center of Baylor College of Medicine in Texas (Frank *et al.*, 1982) compared breast- and bottle-fed infants from that state for their first 6 months. Overall there was no difference in respiratory virus infections, and although there were fewer episodes of bronchiolitis in the breastfed group, the difference was not statistically significant, and both groups used medical care to the same extent.

The systematic review of four trials by Wang and Tang (1999) found that in children born prematurely, in children with bronchopulmonary dys- plasia and in children with a combination of these and other risk factors, prophylactic immunisation with RSV immunoglobulin or monoclonal antibody reduced rates of admission to hospital and intensive care, but there was no reduction in the frequency of mechanical ventilation. Subgroup analysis of the children in these trials found that prophylaxis reduced the number of hospital admissions of children whose only risk factor was prematurity by about 75%, and of those with pulmonary dysplasia alone by about 50%. However, there was no reduction in the number of admissions of children whose only morbidity was cardiac abnormality.

The burden to society caused by RSV infections would be substantially lower if an effective vaccine could be developed. Unfortunately, four decades of work have not yet produced a satisfactory vaccine. Although researchers have been able to stimulate antibody responses in neonatal mice, to date they have been unable to find a vaccine that is effective in immature infants.

Viral bronchiolitis continues to be a major public health problem. Pre- vention of severe RSV-associated bronchiolitis in high-risk infants has been partially achieved by passive administration of humanised mono- clonal antibody. Supportive therapy is the mainstay of treatment. Apart from small and limited groups of at-risk children who may benefit from passive immunoglobulins, there seems to be no effective way of prevent- ing bronchiolitis due to RSV infection in the majority of the child population until a vaccine is developed. Once a child has bronchiolitis, there is no effective cure, and treatment is supportive. The majority of children have only a mild infection, and recover with nursing care alone. Other more severely ill children require oxygen supplementation, intuba- tion and assisted ventilation. The role of the GP, when confronted with a wheezing infant with symptoms of infection (who therefore has bronch- iolitis), is to assess whether the child is seriously ill, or may become so. Not surprisingly, most children with bronchiolitis, even those who are mildly ill, are referred to an inpatient setting for further observation and assessment.

References

Agency for Healthcare Research and Quality (2001) *Management of Bronchiolitis in Infants and Children. Evidence Report/Technology Assessment Number 69.* AHRQ Publication Number 03-E014; www.ahrq.gov/clinic/epcsums/broncsum.htm.

American Academy of Pediatrics, Infectious Diseases Committee (2003) Respiratory syncytial virus. In: LK Pickering (ed.) *Red Book: 2003 Report of the Committee on Infectious Diseases* (26e). American Academy of Pediatrics, Elk Grove Village, IL.

Bordley WC, Viswanathan M, King VJ and Sutton SF (2004) Diagnosis and testing in bronchiolitis: a systematic review. *Arch Pediatr Adol Med.* **158**: 119–26.

Christakis DA, Cowan D, Garrison MM and Colvani R (2005) Variation in inpatient diagnostic testing and management in bronchiolitis. *Pediatrics.* **115**: 878–84.

Everard ML, Bara A, Kurian M, Ellitt TM, Ducharme F and Mayowe V (2001) Anticholinergic drugs for wheeze in children under the age of two years (Cochrane Review). In: *The Cochrane Library. Review CD001279.* Update Software, Oxford.

Flores G and Horwitz RI (1997) Efficacy of beta-2 agonists in bronchiolitis: a reappraisal and meta-analysis. *Pediatrics.* **100**: 233–9.

Frank AL, Taber LH, Glezen WP and Kasel GL (1982) Breast feeding and respiratory virus infection. *Pediatrics.* **72**: 239–45.

Friis B, Andersen P and Brenoe E (1984) Antibiotic treatment of pneumonia and bronchiolitis: a prospective randomized study. *Arch Dis Child.* **59**: 1038–45.

Garrison M, Christakis DA, Harvey E, Cummings P and Davis RL (2000) Systemic corticosteroids in infant bronchiolitis: a meta-analysis. *Pediatrics.* **105**: E44.

Glezen P, Parades A, Allison JE *et al.* (1981) Risk of respiratory syncytial infection in infants from low income families in relationship to age, sex, ethnic group and maternal antibody level. *J Pediatr.* **98**: 708–715.

Goebel L, Estrada B, Quinonez J and Sanford D (2000). Prednisone plus albuterol versus albuterol alone in mild to moderate bronchiolitis. *Clin Pediatr* **29**:213–20.

Gruber W (1997) Bronchiolitis. In: Long S, Pickering I and Prober C (eds). *Principles and Practice of Pediatric Infective Diseases.* Churchill Livingstone, New York.

Hartling L, Wiebe N, Russell K, Patel H and Klassen TP (2001) Epinephrine for bronchiolitis (Cochrane Review). In: *The Cochrane Library. Review CD003123.* Update Software, Oxford.

Kellner JD, Ohlsson A, Gadomski AM and Wang EEL (2001) Bronchodilators for bronchiolitis (Cochrane Review). In: *The Cochrane Library. Review CD001266.* Update Software, Oxford.

King VJ, Viswathanan M, Bordley WC *et al.* (2004) Pharmacologic treatment of bronchiolitis in infants and children: a systematic review. *Arch Pediatr Adolesc Med.* **158**: 127–37.

Klassen TP, Rowe PC, Sutcliffe T and Ropp RJ (1991). Randomized trial of salbutamol in acute bronchiolitis. *J Pediatr* **118**: 807–11.

Langley JM, LeBlanc JC, Smith B and Wang EE (2003). Increasing incidence of hospitalization for bronchiolitis among Canadian children 1980–2000. *J Infect Dis* **188**:1764–7.

McConnaichie KM, Mark JD and McBride JT (1985). Normal pulmonary function measurements and airway reactivity in childhood after mild bronchiolitis. *J Pediatr* **107**: 54–8.

McConnaichie KM and Roughmann KJ (1986). Parental smoking, presence of older siblings and family history increase the risk of bronchiolitis. *Am J Dis Child.* **140**: 806–12.

Navas L, Wang E, de Carvalo V and Robinson J (1992). PICNIC. Improved outcomes of respiratory virus infections in a high-risk hospitalized population of Canadian children. *J Pediatr.* **121**: 348–54.

Patel H, Platt R, Lozano JM and Wang EE (2000) Glucocorticosteroids for acute viral bronchiolitis in infants and young children (Cochrane Review). In: *The Cochrane Library. Review CD004878.* Update Software, Oxford.

Phelan P, Olinsky A and Robertson C (1994). R*espiratory Illness in Children,* 4th edition. Blackwell Scientific Publisher, London.

Randolph AG and Wang EEL (2001) Ribavirin for respiratory syncytial virus lower respiratory tract infection (Cochrane Review). In: *The Cochrane Library. Review CD000181.* Update Software, Oxford.

Reijonen T, Korhonen K and Korrpi M (2000). Predictors of asthma three years after being admitted to hospital with wheezing in infancy. *Pediatrics.* **105**: 13–18.

Sly PD and Hibbert ME (1989). Childhood asthma following hospitalization with acute viral bronchiolitis in infancy. *J Pediatr Pulmonol.* **7**: 153–8.

Steiner RW (2004) Treating acute bronchiolitis associated with RSV. *Am Fam Physician.* **69**: 1101–10.

Tal A, Balvilski C and Yohai D (1983). Dexamethasone and salbutamol in the treatment of acute wheezing infants. *Pediatrics.* **71**:13–18.

Wang EE, Law BJ and Stephens D (1995) PICNIC: Pediatric Investigators Collaborative Network on Infections in Canada study of risk factors and morbidity with RSV disease. *J Pediatr.* **126**: 212–19.

Wang EE, Law BJ, Stevens D and Langley JM (1996). Study of interobserver reliability in clinical assessment of RSV lower respiratory tract infection: a PICNIC study. *Pediatr Pulmonol* **22**: 23–7.

Wang EE and Tang NK (1999) Immunoglobulin for preventing respiratory syncytial virus (Cochrane Review). In: *The Cochrane Library. Review CD001725.* Update Software, Oxford.

van Woensel J and van Aaalderan WM (2002). Bronchiolitis hospitalizations in the Netherlands from 1991–1999. *Arch Dis Child.* **86**: 370–1.

van Woensel J and Kimpen J (2000) Therapy for respiratory tract infections caused by respiratory syncytial virus. *Euro J Paediatrics.* **159**: 391–8.

Chapter 11

Clinical judgement versus diagnostic tests

Errors in judgement must occur in the practice of an art which consists largely in balancing probabilities.

Sir William Osler

The diagnosis of ARIs illustrates well Osler's dictum that 'Medicine is a science of uncertainty and an art of probability.' Only when antibiotics became available, shortly after World War Two, was there a reason for reliably distinguishing between viral and bacterial infection. Unfortunately this is not easy for the acute ARIs, regardless of whether clinical judgement or diagnostic tests are used. It is clear that relying on clinical judgement alone is neither satisfactory nor precise. In Israel, Dr David Lieberman and colleagues compared serological testing of patients with an ARI with physicians' judgements of whether a virus or a bacterium had caused the infection. Clinical judgement was found to have a negative predictive value of 60% and a positive predictive value of only 50%. 'We conclude that physicians' ability to determine whether the infectious aetiology of ARI is viral or bacterial is low, and no more reliable than tossing a coin' (Lieberman *et al.*, 2001).

The uncertainty as to whether an ARI is viral or bacterial affects GPs' prescribing behaviour in a very variable manner. This was first shown in the 1970s, when Dr John Howie conducted a survey of the management of respiratory illness by GPs in Scotland (Howie *et al.*, 1971). He found that the proportion of patients with the clinical diagnosis of 'tonsillitis' ranged from 1% to 47% of all ARIs seen, depending on the GP. More recently, when Dr Jim Hutchinson studied the rates of antibiotic prescribing for ARIs by GPs in Newfoundland (Hutchinson *et al.*, 2001) he found that the rate of diagnosis of bacterial illness ranged from 31% to 66%. A large study conducted by Dr Donald Crombie at the Birmingham Research Unit of the Royal College of General Practitioners (Crombie *et al.*, 1992), which involved 214 524 patients of 115 GPs, confirmed these large variations in diagnosis and prescribing habits. The variations were only marginally attributable to chance, different age, gender and class mix, geographical variation and differences in practice organisation. The investigators concluded that 'Variations in recorded diagnostic rates were mainly due to the consistent but idiosyncratic and selective diagnostic behaviour of doctors' (Crombie *et al.* 1992).

In an ideal world, a constellation of clinical signs, or a single rapid test, would give a precise and reliable diagnosis. In the real world, questions that GPs have to consider include the following.

1 Can clinical features (symptoms and signs) be used to obtain a precise diagnosis?
2 Are diagnostic tests better than clinical judgement?
3 If so, are rapid, reliable and cheap near-patient tests available?
4 Can the tests distinguish between carrier state and infection?

Diagnosis of ARIs in routine general practice is usually clinical, and therapy is usually presumptive. Because of their costs and inconvenience, GPs do not usually use tests. They are aware that laboratory tests for the aetiological agents for ARIs are often insensitive, and that they only identify the causative agent in a minority of cases.

In an attempt to improve the precision of GP diagnosis, much effort has been directed towards the development of ARI clinical decision rules – that is, listings of symptoms and signs which, in certain numbers and combinations, will improve the precision of GP diagnosis. Several sets of decision rules have been produced to help to diagnose acute streptococcal pharyngitis, and rapid tests for use in the GP's surgery have also been developed. Efforts to develop decision rules to aid diagnosis of acute bacterial otitis media and sinusitis have been less successful. Various testing technologies have been advocated for these conditions. With regard to acute bronchitis, the common cold and influenza, diagnosis is almost always clinical (formal rules for these conditions have not been developed, and the traditional diagnostic symptoms and signs are still used). There has been little interest in developing tests for GPs to use for these conditions, although viral tests for influenza are increasingly used by sentinel systems to give an early warning of an approaching epidemic.

In theory, microbiological testing is an important tool for aiding rational prescribing, but in order to be of any use to GPs, the ideal test would have to be quick, cheap, non-invasive and suitable for use in the GP's surgery, giving a result while the patient is still there. If the test results were immediately available, a negative result would make it much easier for the doctor to decline to give an unnecessary antibiotic. If the test result was positive, it might help the GP to decide on the best treatment. Testing in the GP's surgery (or 'near-patient' testing, as it is called in the USA) could also reduce the amount of time that GPs spend filling in forms to accompany specimens to a laboratory, communication problems with the laboratories would no longer exist, and money would be saved on faxes, envelopes and stamps.

Unfortunately, it is by no means certain that making diagnostic tests (even if they are reliable) freely available to GPs will improve the situation. In Denmark, Dr Hans Kolmus (Kolmus *et al.*, 1992) studied what happened when GPs were free to order unlimited tests. Doctors showed 100-fold variation in their rates of ordering tests, and the higher the number of specimens sent in by a doctor, the lower the proportion of positive test results. Another study in Finland, conducted by Dr Henrika Honkanen (Honkanen *et al.*, 2002) looked at the popularity of various ARI tests when they were all available to GPs. Tympanometry was used for only 1% of patients with acute otitis media. Ultrasonography, sinus radiography or both were used in 80% of patients with sinusitis, antigen detection tests were used in 57% of patients with throat infections, and a chest radiograph was taken in only 5% of bronchitis cases. To date, rapid antigen tests for GABHS are only widely used in the USA. Pneumatic otoscopy and tympanometry have not been widely adopted anywhere in primary care settings.

Those who argue against diagnostic testing by GPs point out that even in research studies, micro-organisms are isolated in only 30% of ARI cases. Community laboratories used by GPs would probably have lower isolation rates. Some authors have also questioned whether access to rapid tests will change GPs' behaviour. A study conducted by GPs at the Aldermoor Health Centre in Southampton (Burke, 1988) found that when GPs treated patients with sore throat, they prescribed antibiotics for 64% of them. Then, when the GPs were given access to the results of a rapid enzyme immunoassay test, they changed their prescribing decisions for only 13% of patients. On the other hand, a recent study that I conducted in Newfoundland (Worrall *et al.*, 2005) found that the availability of a rapid antigen test reduced GP antibiotic prescribing from 58% to 27% for adults with sore throat.

More testing will increase the number of patients with false-positive test results, and may increase healthcare spending. Increased use of diagnostic investigations for ARIs would possibly create the impression that it is important for the doctor to do the test. Thus a major cost incurred by diagnostic testing may be that it encourages more testing in patients with self-limiting illness.

Another argument against the use of microbiological testing for ARIs in the community is the high rate of carriage of potentially pathogenic bacteria such as *Streptococcus pneumoniae* and *Haemophilus influenzae*. Children in particular appear to have high rates of carriage, up to 50%. Recovery of pathogenic bacteria from purulent nasopharyngitis specimens is almost always due to carriage rather than infection. Most infectious disease experts would not accept that isolation of a bacterial 'pathogen' from the nose of a patient with a common cold is an indication of bacterial infection. Furthermore, in patients with a positive throat culture, serological evidence of recent infection is found in only 20–50% of cases. Clearly, a high proportion of bacterial isolates represent the carrier state in individuals who are probably in fact suffering from a viral infection.

Tests for specific ARIs

Colds
No testing is needed.
Always a clinical diagnosis.

Sore throats
Use validated decision rules.
Consider an antigen test in doubtful cases.

Otitis media
Usually a clinical diagnosis.
No clear decision rules.
Consider pneumatic otoscopy.

Bronchitis
Usually a clinical diagnosis.
No clear decision rules.
No definitive test.

Sinusitis
Usually a clinical diagnosis.
No clear decision rules.
No definitive test.

Influenza
Usually a clinical diagnosis.
Testing is for public health reasons only.

Croup
Always a clinical diagnosis.

Bronchiolitis
Always a clinical diagnosis.

Common cold

The common cold is always a clinical diagnosis, often by the patient, and rarely contradicted by the physician. As there are over 200 known viral causative agents, testing is not necessary unless the GP suspects that something more serious is going on. A study of people aged 60–90 years living in the UK (Nicholson *et al.*, 1997) found that a causative agent could be isolated in only 43% of cases. Of the identified organisms, 52% were rhinoviruses and 26% were coronaviruses. There was no pathognomic feature for any one organism. In younger people, a study of 200 university students with common colds in Turku, Finland (Makela *et al.*, 1998) was able to isolate a virus in 69% of cases. Once again, rhinoviruses were most commonly identified, representing 76% of isolates.

Acute sore throat

The identification and treatment of GABHS infection in people with sore throats was once considered important because it was believed that treatment promotes the resolution of symptoms (resulting in fewer days lost from school or work), reduces the severity of symptoms, shortens the duration of infectivity, reduces the spread of illness, prevents the development of acute respiratory failure and decreases the incidence of suppurative complications. Recent reviews of the evidence have indicated that these benefits are marginal at best (Del Mar, 2004; ICSI, 2004). The development and use of decision rules for sore throat has mitigated against the use of testing for GABHS in general practice. The early antigen tests took several hours to complete, but recent GP surgery tests based on optical immunoassay can give a result (shown as a change in a coloured strip) within 5 minutes. These tests perform slightly better than the older antigen tests and the traditional agar cultures, with a sensitivity and specificity greater than 90%. Most authorities now recommend that these tests be used judiciously, in combination with clinical decision rules.

Acute otitis media

As nasopharyngeal cultures do not accurately predict the bacteriology of middle ear infection, and culture of middle ear aspirate is not possible unless the eardrum is perforated, an array of gadgets has been used to test for ear infections. Pneumatic otoscopy, which is sensitive to immobility of the tympanum, has proved very useful in ENT clinic studies, but its value in the primary care setting, where serious infection of the middle ear is much less common, is not known. There are no published studies that have compared regular with pneumatic otoscopy in the general practice environment. Tympanometry and acoustic reflectometry have been used in research studies, but are unlikely to find a place in general practice (Coombs, 1994). Although there are no formal decision rules for acute otitis media, the positive predictive values of physical findings for this condition are as follows: bulging tympanic membrane, 89%; cloudy tympanic membrane, 80%; impaired mobility, 78%. If more than one of these signs is present, the positive predictive value for diagnosis of acute otitis media is greater than 90% (Karma *et al.*, 1989).

Acute bronchitis

Bronchitis is difficult to diagnose, although many GPs do so confidently. Although it is known that respiratory viruses cause about 85% of cases of acute bronchitis, it is difficult to isolate the micro-organism. Even when bacteria are isolated from the sputum of people with acute bronchitis, their role is difficult to assess because of the high rates of oropharyngeal colonisation in healthy individuals. Several studies have shown that GPs differ widely in the criteria that they use to diagnose 'bronchitis'. The strongest positive predictors were cough, wheezing, older age, cigarette smoking, a history of previous bronchitis, and being seen by an older GP. There are no valid decision rules for bronchitis. It has been suggested that pulmonary function tests are helpful for diagnosing acute bronchitis. In a study of American family practice by Dr Harold Williamson (Williamson, 1987) of the patients who were diagnosed with bronchitis, 40% had an FEV1 value that was less than 80% of normal. Since there is no gold-standard test, the diagnosis of acute bronchitis must be made on clinical grounds. The usual criteria are purulent cough of less than 2 weeks' duration, no history of previous lung disease, and the absence of clinical evidence of pneumonia and asthma.

Acute sinusitis

The diagnosis and treatment of bacterial sinusitis are confusing to physicians for several reasons. Its presentation is similar to that of viral upper respiratory tract infection, an easy-to-use diagnostic test is lacking, and the gold standard – sinus aspiration and culture – cannot be performed in daily clinical practice. Several studies have evaluated the symptoms and signs compared with a CT scan diagnosis of bacterial sinusitis. The appropriately named Sino-Nasal Outcome Test (SNOT), performed by Dr Tammy Bhattacharyya and colleagues in Boston (Bhattacharya *et al.*, 1997) compared the responses of 221 patients to a 20-item questionnaire with CT scans. The most commonly reported symptoms were fatigue and sinus pain or pressure, and there was little correlation between symptoms and CT scan results. Also comparing CT scan results with clinical diagnosis, a study by Lindbaek *et al.* (1996) of 201 primary care patients in Norway found that the presence of three out of four variables (three signs and one blood test) was associated with a sensitivity of 60% and a specificity of 81% for predicting sinusitis. A study that used antral puncture as the gold standard found that positive clinical examination, combined with either a positive radiograph or ultrasound examination, was the best diagnostic combination, giving a sensitivity of 58% and a specificity of 88% (De Bock, 1994). Several studies have found that CT scans of the sinuses are of limited diagnostic value – they may be no better than plain radiography. Although CT scanning is now regarded as the gold standard of sinus imaging, the soft tissue changes that it often shows so clearly do not correlate well with the major signs and symptoms of sinusitis. CT scanning cannot distinguish between bacterial sinusitis and viral infection, and it often detects mucosal thickening in people with the common cold, and even in asymptomatic individuals. Furthermore, many people with antrally diagnosed sinusitis have negative CT scans. Imaging studies are not currently recommended for the routine diagnosis of uncomplicated sinusitis presenting to the GP.

Influenza

Several general practice studies have tried to develop the clinical model that will best predict the presence of influenza. A study by van Elden *et al.* (2001) in the Netherlands found that the symptom combination of fever, cough and headache during the influenza season had a positive predictive value of 75%. In Canada, Dr Guy Boivin's study of 100 adults with flu-like illness (Boivin *et al.*, 2002) found that a combination of fever plus two out of four symptoms (cough, myalgia, sore throat and headache) had a sensitivity of 78%, a specificity of 55% and a positive predictive value of 87% for influenza. In the USA, Dr Arnold Monto and colleagues (Monto *et al.*, 2000) used multivariate analysis to develop the optimal clinical predictive model for influenza. Once again fever and cough were the best predictors. Fever and two of the same four symptoms that were used in the Canadian study had a sensitivity of 64%, a specificity of 67% and a positive predictive value of 79% for influenza.

The traditional techniques for confirming influenza infection (culture and serology) take several days to complete. Some recent polymerase chain reaction tests will detect influenza A only, others will detect A or B, and yet others can distinguish between A and B. They take only 30 minutes to complete. As these virological tests are very expensive, they will clearly not be used in day-to-day practice, where the reliance on clinical judgement will continue, with some GPs doing tests so that they can inform the public health authorities when a new epidemic of influenza is beginning (Carman *et al.*, 2000).

Croup

This is always a clinical diagnosis for GPs. Viral cultures have only been used in research studies.

Bronchiolitis

This is also a clinical diagnosis in primary care.

Thus it is clear that ARIs are usually diagnosed clinically, even when fairly reliable tests, such as those for streptococcal antigen, are available. Testing has not become common because it is expensive and inconvenient, and because GPs, rightly or wrongly, trust their own clinical judgement. Testing can only be justified if it is felt that GPs' judgment is poor, and that the consequences of an incorrect clinical decision by the GP would be very serious. The justification for testing has been that it helps to target treatment. Even if the tests were perfect, and we had universally effective treatments, would better diagnosis lead to an appreciable health gain? The ARIs are usually short-term and self-limiting conditions, and the need to diagnose the organism responsible is therefore questionable. The only probable justification for most acute ARIs is that the tests may result in lower rates of antibiotic prescribing.

With regard to preventing the rare complications of the ARIs, we in primary care have little idea whether better microbiological diagnosis is the key, or whether it is more important to identify clinical or socio-demographic subgroups that are at risk. Unfortunately, very large and expensive clinical trials would need to be conducted in the low-prevalence primary care setting in order to generate unbiased clinical and micro-biological answers, and such studies will probably never be done. In the mean time, if we make the generous assumption that every complication is preventable, we would have to test hundreds of people in order to prevent even the most common non-life-threatening complications, such as quinsy.

References

Bhattacharya T, Picinnillo J and Wippold F (1997) Relationship between patient-based descriptions of sinusitis and paranasal CT findings. *Arch Laryngol Head Neck Surg.* **123**: 1189–92.

Boivin G, Hardy I, Tellier LL and Maziade J (2002) Predicting influenza infection during epidemics with the use of a clinical case definition. *Clin Infect Dis.* **31**: 1166–9.

Burke P, Bain J, Lowes AM and Athersuch R (1988). Rational decisions in managing sore throat: evaluation of a rapid test. *BMJ.* **296**: 1646–9.

Carman WF, Wallace LA, Walker J *et al.* (2000) Rapid virological surveillance of community influenza infection in general practice. *BMJ.* **321**: 736–7.

Coombs JT (1994) The diagnosis of otitis media: new techniques. *Pediatr Infect Dis J.* **13**: 1046–9.

Crombie DL, Cross KW and Fleming DM (1992) The problem of diagnostic variability in general practice. *J Epidemiol Comm Health.* **46**: 447–54.

De Bock GH, Houwing-Duistermatt JJ, Springer MP *et al.* (1994). Sensitivity and specificity of diagnostic tests in acute maxillary sinusitis in the absence of a diagnostic standard. *J Clin Epidemiol.* **47**: 1343–52.

Del Mar C, Glasziou P and Spinks AB. (2001) Antibiotics for sore throat (Cochrane Review). In: *The Cochrane Library. Review CD000023.*

Gerber M (1989) Comparison of throat cultures and rapid Strep tests for the diagnosis of streptococcal pharyngitis. *Pediatr Infect Dis J.* **8**: 820–24.

Howie JG, Richardson IM, Gill G and Durno D (1971) Respiratory illness and antibiotic use in general practice. *Roy Coll GP J.* **21**: 657–61

Honkanen PO, Rautakorpi UM, Huovinen P, Klaukka T, *et al.* (2002) Diagnostic tools in respiratory tract infections: use and comparison with Finnish guidelines. *Scand J Inf Dis.* **34**: 827–30.

Hutchinson JM, Jelinsky S, Hefferton E, *et al.* (2001) Role of diagnostic labeling in antibiotic prescription. *Can Fam Phys.* **47**: 1217–24.

Institute for Clinical Systems Improvement. (2001) *Health Care Guideline: Acute Pharyngitis. General Implementation.* www.icsi.org.

Karma PH, Penttila MA, Kataja MD and Sipila MM (1989) Otoscopic diagnosis of middle ear effusion in acute and non-acute otitis media. *Int J Ped Otolarygol.* **17**: 37–49.

Kolmus HJ, Kgaeldgaard P and Jensen K (1992) Clinical microbiological service in primary health care in the municipality of Copenhagen. *Ugeskr Laeger.* **154**: 2810–14.

Lieberman D, Schvartzman P, Korsorsky I and Lieberman D (2001) Aetiology of respiratory tract infections: clinical assessment versus serological tests. *Br J Gen Pract.* **51**: 999–1000.

Lindbaek M, Hjortdahl P and Johnsen ULH (1996) Use of symptoms, signs, and blood tests to diagnose sinusitis: comparison with CT. *Fam Med.* **28**: 183–8.

Makela A, Puhakka T, Ruuskanen O, *et al.* 1998). Viruses and bacteria in the aetiology of the common cold. *J Clin Microbiol.* **36**: 539–42.

Monto AS, Gravenstein AS, Elliott M, *et al.* (2000) Clinical signs and symptoms predicting influenza infection. *Arch Int Med.* **116**: 3242–7.

Nicholson KG, Kent J, Hammersley V and Cancio E (1997). Acute viral infections of the upper respiratory tract in elderly people living in the community: comparative prospective population-based study of disease burden. *BMJ.* **315**: 1060–4.

van Elden LJ, van Essen GA, Boucher CA *et al.* (2001) Clinical diagnosis of influenza virus infection: evaluation of diagnostic tools in general practice. *Br J Gen Pract.* **51**: 630–34.

Williamson HA. (1987) Pulmonary function tests in acute bronchitis: evidence for reversible airway obstruction. *J Fam Pract.* **25**: 251–7.

Worrall G, Sherman G, Hutchinson J (2005) A randomized trial of in-office aids to help of diagnosis of streptococcal sore throat in primary care. Canadian College of Family Practice Forum, Vancouver, September.

Chapter 12

Antibiotic prescribing and resistance

One of the first duties of the physician is to educate the masses not to take medicine.

Sir William Osler

- Since penicillin was introduced in the 1940s, antibiotic use has exploded throughout the world.
- After the introduction of a new antibiotic, resistant organisms soon appear.
- Factors that encourage antibiotic resistance include the following:
  - widespread use in livestock
  - widespread use in humans, especially children
  - increased travel
  - increased GP prescribing.
- Some countries have been able to reduce antibiotic resistance by changing antibiotic-prescribing policies.

In February 1941, a young policeman in Oxford, England developed severe cellulitis after scratching his face on a rose bush. Dr Howard Florey and his colleagues made medical history by treating the patient with intravenous penicillin. The patient at first showed a remarkable improvement, but after 5 days the physicians' tiny supply of the antibiotic ran out. The patient relapsed and died 10 days later. Despite this tragic result, the antibiotic era had begun.

In the following two decades, it become apparent that doctors in general, and GPs in particular, were extremely fond of these antimicrobial agents and were very willing to prescribe them, even for illnesses that were almost certainly viral in origin. There was an innocent worldwide expectation that infectious diseases would be conquered. This optimism was soon quenched by the emergence of penicillin-resistant *Staphylococcus aureus*. By 1946, 90% of staphylococci found in hospitals were already resistant to penicillin (Finland, 1955). The great influenza pandemic of 1957–58 was associated with a simultaneous outbreak of penicillin-resistant *S. aureus* phage type 80/81, following the prescribing of penicillin for the illness.

Resistance to tetracycline was first reported in 1963, followed by reports of resistance to penicillin and erythromycin in 1967. When an organism develops resistance to penicillin, it often also becomes resistant to other antibiotics. During succeeding decades, the introduction of numerous antibiotic agents was followed – inevitably, it seemed – by the emergence of resistance among many bacterial species. This pattern of discovery, exuberant use and development of resistance was repeated after the introduction of each new antibiotic. No collective memory of the recent past seemed to exist in the medical profession. Vast amounts of antibiotics were produced and consumed globally; in 1980, 15.5 million kilograms of penicillin were produced, which is the equivalent of 3.85 grams for each person on the planet (Cole and O'Connor, 1987). In addition to the widespread use of antibiotics by humans, and the effect that this has in selecting resistant bacteria, there is also evidence that excess consumption of antibiotics by domesticated livestock is contributing to the emergence of resistance. At the present time, livestock and poultry consume approximately 40% of the antibiotics produced in the USA (Institute of Medicine, 1989). Antibiotic pressure on bacterial organisms creates a situation of 'survival of the fittest', with elimination of the most susceptible competitors. Studies in the USA, Iceland, Spain, France, Hungary and South Africa, as well as in the UK, have shown a correlation between antibiotic use and the development of resistant strains of *Streptococcus pneumoniae*.

Paediatric studies have found that children who have recently taken antibiotics show a two- to sevenfold increase in the likelihood that they will become colonised with resistant organisms compared with children who have not received antibiotics (Jackson *et al.*, 1984; Brook and Gober, 1996). Once antibiotic resistance has developed in an individual, transmission of the resistant strain to close contacts occurs. Many studies have shown that children in day-care centres have increased levels of resistant bacteria. In a study of American children with recurrent otitis media (Nyquist *et al.*, 1998), those children who were given antibiotics as prophylaxis all carried antibiotic-resistant organisms after 5 months. Fortunately, the proportion of resistant organisms decreased once the prophylactic therapy was discontinued. A more recent study, by Dr Dilruba Nasrin (Nasrin *et al.*, 2002), followed Australian preschool children prospectively for 25 months. The likelihood of carrying penicillin-resistant pneumococci was doubled in children who had received one beta-lactam (such as a penicillin or a cephalosporin) in the preceding 2 months, and quadrupled in children who had taken two beta-lactams. Those who had taken antibiotics for more than 2 weeks in the preceding 6 months were twice as likely to have penicillin-resistant pneumococci as those who had received antibiotics for 1 week or less. The likelihood of carrying resistant micro-organisms increased by 4% for every day of antibiotic consumption in the previous 6 months.

Worldwide travel is helping to spread antibiotic-resistant bacteria. In an elegant study (Soares, 1993) a team at Rockefeller University presented convincing evidence that a single multi-resistant *S. pneumoniae* clone had been imported into Iceland from Spain, presumably by returning holiday-makers. Those researchers found evidence of the global spread of antibiotic-resistant organisms when the same resistance clone was identified in samples from Spain, the USA, Mexico, Portugal, France, Croatia and South Africa.

It seems clear that the excessive use of antibiotics in ambulatory practice by GPs has contributed to the emergence and spread of antibiotic-resistant bacteria in the community. Recent reports indicate that over 40% of *S. pneumoniae* isolates in carriers are non-susceptible to penicillin (Kunin, 1993; Barry *et al.*, 1994). A consistent finding of these reports is that the most important risk factor for transmission of and infection with resistant organisms is current or recent antibiotic use. Antibiotic use in the previous 3 to 6 months has been linked with a two- to fivefold increase in the risk of nasopharyngeal colonisation with antibiotic-resistant *S. pneumoniae* (Brook and Gober, 1996). The risk of sepsis and meningitis due to antibiotic-resistant pneumococci was increased substantially following exposure to antibiotics; in a case–control study conducted by Dr James Kellner and the Toronto Child Care Study Group, it was demonstrated that children with invasive antibiotic-resistant pneumococcal infections were 3.5 times more likely to have received a course of antibiotics in the previous month than children with infections due to susceptible pneumococci (Kellner and Ford-Jones, 1999). In a prospective population-based cohort study conducted by Dr Juan Nava on individuals from an industrial suburb of Barcelona, Spain, 23.5% of patients were found to be infected with penicillin-resistant *S. pneumoniae* (Nava *et al.*, 1994). Resistant organisms were more commonly found in children under 5 years of age, and were strongly associated with previous recent use of a beta-lactam. A study of adults with pneumonia, conducted by Dr Calvin Kunin in the USA found that one-third of patients were infected with antibiotic-resistant organisms (Kunin, 1993). The death rate was much higher (54%) in people infected with resistant pneumococci than in those with penicillin-sensitive organisms (25%). A study conducted in Perth, Australia, by Dr John Turnidge and colleagues found that 25.4% of all bacteria were resistant to penicillin, 15.7% were resistant to tetracycline, 15.6% were resistant to erythromycin and 21.2% were resistant to more than one antibiotic (Turnidge, 1999). Similar patterns of emerging resistance have been found in other countries.

Streptococcus pyogenes continues to remain exquisitely sensitive to penicillin, because of its inability to produce beta-lactamase. In contrast, resistance of *Haemophilus influenzae* to ampicillin was described as early as 1974, and is now thought to occur in 35% of cases. Once thought to be a harmless respiratory tract commensal, *Moraxella catarrhalis* is a respiratory pathogen in the elderly and a causative agent of sinusitis and otitis media in children. The first report of a beta-lactamase-producing strain of *M. catarrhalis* appeared in 1976 (Kunin, 1993), and now 90% of *M. catarrhalis* produces beta-lactamase. Macrolide resistance appears to develop faster than resistance to other antibiotics. By the late 1970s 60% of *S. pyogenes* in Japan had become resistant to erythromycin.

Can anything be done about antibiotic resistance? Fortunately, the continued emergence of antibiotic resistance need not be inevitable. Several countries have shown that enlightened national policies on antibiotic use can reduce resistance rates and thus provide an effective public health response to the problem. In Japan in the mid-1970s, the level of erythromycin use was very high, and erythromycin resistance of *S. pyogenes* reached an all-time high of 61.4%. By the mid-1980s, when the prescribing of erythromycin had decreased to less than half the former amount, erythromycin resistance had decreased to 1–3%. The same phenomenon was observed in Finland, where in the 1980s the consumption of erythromycin almost tripled, and resistant organisms emerged. The Finnish medical authorities responded by issuing nationwide recommendations to reduce macrolide prescribing for outpatients. The percentage of resistant strains of *S. pyogenes* decreased from 16.5% in 1992 to 8.6% in 1996 (Seppala *et al.*, 1997). Similarly, in Hungary there was a steady drop in the level of penicillin-resistant *S. pneumoniae*, associated with a major reduction in the use of penicillin (Nowak, 1994). In Iceland there were similar declines in the mid-1990s following a decrease in the overall number of antibiotics prescribed (Kristinsson, 1997).

There is less antibiotic resistance in the Netherlands than in other European countries. This is probably due to a long-standing culture of low antibiotic prescribing, reflected in the guidelines for the management of acute ARIs produced by the Royal Dutch College of General Practice (De Neeling *et al.*, 1993) which emphasise the viral nature of most such illnesses, and the efficacy of a watch-and-wait strategy for these mostly self-limiting diseases.

General practitioners can be described as being addicted to the prescribing of antibiotics. By the 1970s, Dr John Howie found that GPs in the UK were prescribing antibiotics for 75% of ARIs (Howie and Hutchinson, 1978). In the 1980s, when Canadian GPs were shown case vignettes of patients with ARIs in a study by Stephenson *et al.* (1988), they indicated that they would prescribe antibiotics 50% of the time. Similarly, a study of Danish GPs in 1987, conducted by Dr Henrik Friis (Friis *et al.*, 1989) found that they prescribed antibiotics for 75% of upper respiratory tract infections.

It would be nice to think that all of the evidence mentioned in the previous chapters – that ARIs are mostly viral in origin and that, even

- All over the world, GPs have high antibiotic-prescribing rates.
- There is wide variation in antibiotic-prescribing rates between countries.
- Within countries, there is wide variation in antibiotic-prescribing rates between individual doctors.
- There are a number of different reasons why GPs prescribe 'against the evidence':
  - they wish to fulfil perceived patient expectations
  - older doctors prescribe more
  - fee-for-service doctors prescribe more
  - busy doctors prescribe more
  - doctors are not concerned about resistant organisms developing.
- Diagnostic labelling is thought to justify many antibiotic prescriptions.

when due to bacteria, they are mostly mild and self-limiting illnesses, for which the administration of antibiotics produces only minimal reductions in severity and duration of symptoms – would have caused a stampede away from liberal antibiotic use.

However, by the late 1990s not much had changed – 87% of people with a cough were still given antibiotics by GPs in the UK. An interesting study by Cars *et al.* (2001) compared non-hospital antibiotic sales in 15 member states of the European Union. It was found that sales varied by more than fourfold from country to country. France, Spain, Portugal and Belgium had the highest sales, and the Netherlands, Denmark, Sweden and Germany had the lowest.

Across the Atlantic in the USA, the condition for which antibiotics were most frequently used in the outpatient setting was acute otitis media. Antibiotic prescriptions for this diagnosis increased from 12 million in 1980 to 24 million in 1992 (McCaig and Hughes, 1995; Gonzales *et al.*, 1997). The 1992 National Ambulatory Care Survey found that antibiotics were also frequently prescribed for adults for colds, upper respiratory tract infections and bronchitis (three illnesses of viral aetiology) (NAMCS, 1994). ARIs were responsible for 33% of all GP antimicrobial prescribing. Around 51% of patients with colds and 66% of those with bronchitis were prescribed antibiotics. In the USA, Nyquist *et al.* (1998) found that in paediatric practice, children aged 0–4 years received 53% of all antibiotics prescribed, and 30% of all antibiotics prescribed for children were for acute otitis media. Doctors prescribed antibiotics for 44% of children with colds and 75% of children with bronchitis. North of the border, Dr Jim Hutchinson found that 75% of antibiotic prescriptions given by Canadian GPs were for respiratory tract disease (Hutchinson and Foley, 1999).

The situation was much the same in Australia (Nasrin *et al.*, 2002). In a prospective study of preschool children in Canberra, Dr Nasrin's group found that 47% of all episodes of ARI resulted in a visit to the doctor, and 48% of children who saw the doctor received an antibiotic prescription at the first visit (Nasrin, 2002).

Outside the European Union, in Finland, 74% of all antibiotic pre-scriptions were for acute ARIs (Rautakorpi *et al.*, 2001). In Danish general practice, 87% of patients with acute bronchitis were prescribed antibiotics (Friis *et al.*, 1989). In Croatia, 66% of ARI cases were prescribed antibiotics, even in university teaching practices (Cars *et al.*, 2001)

Thus it seems clear that there has been little change in the prescribing behaviour of GPs, despite good evidence that antibiotics are not an effective treatment for most ARIs. In theory, the evidence makes it possible for a GP to say to a patient, once an ARI has been diagnosed, something along the following lines: 'You have a 75–85% chance of feeling better within 7–11 days, without treatment. If I give you anti-biotics, there may be a slight improvement, but it is so slight that I would have to treat nine people like you for one to benefit, and I don't know whether you will be one of the eight who will get no benefit. And by the way, one out of 15 people who take the antibiotic experience unpleasant side-effects. Do you still wish to take it?'

One of the great conundrums of primary care is why the prescribing of ineffective antibiotics continues. Researchers have scratched their heads and attempted to discover why GPs in all countries seem to be 'prescribing against the evidence.'

A study of primary care paediatricians in the USA by Dr Rebecca Watson (Watson *et al.*, 1999) found that although 97% of doctors agreed that overuse of antibiotics is a major factor in the development of antibiotic resistance, and that they should therefore be prescribed judiciously, actual behaviours were different. In total, 69% of respondents considered purulent rhinitis to be a diagnostic finding that required antibiotics, 86% prescribed antibiotics for bronchitis regardless of the duration of the cough, and 42% prescribed antibiotics for the common cold. Another study in the USA, conducted by Dr David Vinson (Vinson and Lutz, 1993) found that even when doctors knew about the possibility that excess prescribing caused antibacterial resistance, they still prescribed antibiotics for children when parents believed that the treatment would be beneficial. A qualitative study conducted by Dr Samuel Coenen (Coenen *et al.*, 2000) revealed similar attitudes among GPs in Belgium.

A survey by Dr Christopher Butler and colleagues at the University of Wales in Cardiff (Butler *et al.*, 1998) found that GPs thought many patients expected an antibiotic and, as most doctors believed that the use of antibiotics presents minimal risks, and did not wish to risk losing patient loyalty, they acceded to this demand. Doctors knew of the evidence for the marginal effectiveness of antibiotics, yet often prescribed them in order to ensure the maintenance of good relationships with patients. For the GPs, possible patient benefit was considered to outweigh theoretical community risk due to resistant bacteria. However, most doctors found prescribing 'against the evidence' an uncomfortable experience.

Another study by Dr Jim Hutchinson (Hutchinson and Foley, 1999), which evaluated all antibiotic prescriptions generated by GPs in Newfoundland over a 1-year period, found that fee-for-service payment and higher volume of patients were strongly associated with higher antibiotic-prescribing rates. Older physicians prescribed more antibiotics than did younger ones. In a study conducted in Denmark, Dr Henrik Friis examined the effect of a reduction in reimbursement on the use of antibiotics by GPs (Friis *et al.*, 1993). When doctors were paid less for writing antibiotic prescriptions, the level of prescribing decreased. GPs in the UK and the Netherlands (who work under a capitation or salaried system) prescribed fewer antibiotics than did fee-for-service GPs in Belgium and North America.

In a study by Britten and Ukoumunne (1997) of patients attending GPs in London, it was found that 'Doctors' perceptions of patients' hope was the strongest influence affecting prescribing.' Similarly, a study of patients with sore throat in Australia, by Dr Kenneth Thomas (Thomas, 1978) found that when the GP thought the patient expected medication, the patient was ten times more likely to get it. The doctor's opinion about the patient's expectation was by far the strongest determinant of prescribing.

Doctors often relate their antibiotic-prescribing decisions to clinical symptoms and signs of dubious diagnostic value. A study of doctor-related variables that predicted antibiotic prescribing in general practice in the USA (Dosh *et al.*, 2000) found that sinus tenderness, added lung sounds, discoloured nasal discharge and post-nasal drainage were all associated with increased antibiotic prescribing. In Queensland, 20 Australian GPs participated in a study by Dr Simon Murray (Murray *et al.*, 2000) and responded to hypothetical clinical vignettes of a 20-year-old patient with an ARI. It was found that doctors were more likely to prescribe antibiotics when there was cough producing yellow sputum, presence of sore throat, fever, or coloured nasal mucus. The investigators concluded that GPs' decisions to prescribe antibiotics were influenced by 'Clinical symptoms and signs for which there is poor evidence for antibiotic efficacy in the literature.'

In Belgium, Dr Samuel Coenen and colleagues (Coenen *et al.*, 2002) ran discussion groups with GPs, to explain their diagnostic and therapeutic decisions with regard to adults who had a cough. Doctors said that prescribing antibiotics unnecessarily was less inappropriate than inappro-priately not prescribing antibiotics. They were strongly influenced by patients' expectation of an antibiotic. Finally, if a GP had had a previous negative experience of not prescribing antibiotics (i.e. the doctor had failed to prescribe them, and the patient become more ill), they were much more likely to prescribe now. Another study by the same investigators (Van Duijin et al., 2003) looked at predictors of antibiotic treatment by GPs for patients with 'sinusitis.' By far the strongest independent predictor was not a clinical symptom or sign, but the prescribing rate (or habit) of the individual doctor.

Diagnostic labelling occurs when a doctor attaches a name to a patient's complaint in order to either justify or make the doctor feel more comfortable with their prescribing behaviour. This has been identified as a particular problem with the ARIs. Doctors may say that a patient has 'bronchitis' or 'sinusitis' rather than a 'chest cold' or a 'head cold', and then offer antibiotics. A retrospective review of patients with 'acute sinusitis' and 'ARI', undertaken in the USA (Hueston et al., 1998) found that there was very little clinical difference between the two groups, but that a far higher proportion of the 'acute sinusitis' patients were prescribed antibiotics. The Newfoundland GP study conducted by Dr Jim Hutchinson (Hutchinson et al., 2001) found that some were 'low prescribers' and some were 'high prescribers.' Although the doctors were of similar age, and saw similar patients, with similar presenting complaints, the 'high prescribers' diagnosed bacterial ARIs in 65.4% of cases, whereas the 'low prescribers' diagnosed bacterial infections in 31.0% of patients. In Belgium, Dr Coenen's group found that the diagnosis of 'sinusitis' or 'sinus tenderness' increased the rate of antibiotic prescribing by fourfold, whereas the label 'flu-like illness' decreased the rate of antibiotic prescribing by tenfold (Coenen et al., 2002) Similarly, in the Netherlands, a study of GPs by Dr Jan de Maeseneer found that the diagnosis of 'sinusitis' was associated with antibiotic prescribing but the diagnosis of 'flu-like illness' was not (de Maeseneer, 1990). In the USA, a study of children attending general practices by Dr Daniel Vinson found that a diagnosis of 'bronchitis' doubled the rate of antibiotic prescribing, whereas a diagnosis of 'viral upper respiratory infection' decreased it by half (Vinson and Lutz, 1993). Diagnostic labelling occurs in all primary care settings.

Is the profligate use of antibiotics entirely the fault of the GPs? Once, while driving along the freeway, I was listening to a phone-in radio show. One caller was irate that her GP had not prescribed an antibiotic, but had only offered her advice. She thought that she should not pay for that visit! The radio show host asked for callers to comment on this. Nine out of the next ten callers agreed that this patient had definitely not been given value for her money.

This brought home to me the idea that perhaps GPs should not be given all the blame for excessive antibiotic use. Many patients really do believe that antibiotics are the most effective treatment for ARIs. A survey of patients in nine European countries found that 87% of them believed that antibiotics were useful for ARIs (Pechere, 2001). Another survey in the USA found that 79% of respondents expected to be given an antibiotic for an ARI (Mainous *et al.*, 1997). Whether real or perceived, patients' expectations concerning antibiotics affect doctors' prescribing behaviour. In Australia, it has been found that if the GP thinks the patient expects an antibiotic, the patient is ten times more likely to be given one (Thomas, 1978) and in Belgium the patient was five times more likely to be given an antibiotic if they expected one (Coenen *et al.*, 2000). In these studies, a high rate of antibiotic prescribing was related to higher overall patient satisfaction with their visit to the GP.

However, there is also some evidence that patients want more than automatic prescriptions when they see their doctor. Dr Butler's team interviewed patients who had recently consulted their GP about a sore throat (Butler *et al.*, 1998). Only a third of these patients had clear expectations that they would be given antibiotics (and usually received them), while the other two-thirds did not. For example, mothers were more likely to accept non-antibiotic treatment for their children than for themselves. Patient satisfaction was not necessarily related to receiving antibiotics – many people were looking for reassurance, further informa-tion and pain relief. A focus group run by the Australian National Prescribing Service found that most patients would rather be given a firm diagnosis and reassurance than an antibiotic (NPS News, 2002), while a survey conducted in the USA by Dr Robert Hamm of Oklahoma found that patient satisfaction was no higher when antibiotics were prescribed than when they were not (Hamm *et al.*, 1996). Patients attending GPs in London were administered a Patient Expectation Questionnaire while they were waiting to see the doctor (Williams *et al.*, 1995). The most widely expected item was 'explanation of the problem', and there was much less demand for 'support' or 'tests and diagnosis.' Patients who had more of their expectations met were more satisfied. A large survey, conducted on over 3000 patients in eight European countries (Grol and Wensing, 1999), found that patients ranked getting enough time with their GP and receiving enough information about their illness as their highest priorities.

Is there any good news on the antibiotic front? In some countries, there is evidence of a recent slight decline in antibiotic prescribing. In the USA, between 1989–90 and 1999–2000 there was an overall decrease of 30% in antibiotic prescribing rates for the five commonest respiratory complaints (McCaig *et al.*, 2002). Another US study found that although between 1991 and 1999 antibiotics were less frequently used for the common cold and pharyngitis, the use of broad-spectrum agents increased from 24% to

48% of antibiotic prescriptions for adults, and from 23% to 40% of those for children (Steinman *et al.*, 2003). In England, there was a 25% decrease in antibiotic prescribing by GPs between 1995 and 2000, the largest reductions being in prescribing rates for children (Majeed and Wrigley, 2002). However, the situation does not appear so rosy elsewhere. Of the countries in the European Union, seven showed an increase in antibiotic use between 1993 and 1997, with the largest increases occurring in Italy (34%) and Luxembourg (12%). Five countries showed a decrease in antibiotic use, with the largest decrease (22%) occurring in Sweden. In France, the number of ARIs that were treated with antibiotics increased by 86% for adults and by 115% for children during the period 1981–92 (Cars *et al.*, 2001).

Years of prescribing and taking antibiotics for viral respiratory infections have created a cycle of supply and demand, reinforcing behaviours that are ineffective. The breaking of this cycle will require educating the public that past practices are no longer optimal, and convincing physicians that a patient's satisfaction is based more on communication than on prescription.

References

Barry AL, Pfaller MA, Fuchs PC and Packer RR (1994) In-vitro activities of twelve orally administered antimicrobial agents against four species of bacterial respiratory pathogens from US medical centres 1992–1993. *Antimicrob Agents Chemotherapy.* **38**: 2419–25.

Britten N and Ukoumunne O (1997) The influence of patients' hopes of receiving a prescription on doctors' perceptions and the decision to prescribe: a questionnaire study. *BMJ.* **315**: 1506–10.

Brook I and Grober AE (1996) Prophylaxis with amoxycillin or sufasoxazole for otitis media: effect on the recovery of penicillin-resistant bacteria from children. *Clin Infect Dis.* **22**: 143–5.

Butler CC, Rollnick S, Pill R, Maggs-Rapport F and Stott N (1998) Understanding the culture of prescribing: qualitative study of general practitioners' and patients' perceptions of antibiotics for sore throats. *BMJ.* **317**: 637–42.

Cars O, Molstad S and Melander A (2001) Variation in antibiotic use in the European Union. *Lancet.* **357**: 1851–3.

Coenen S, Michiels B, Van Royen P *et al.* (2002). Antibiotics for coughing in general practice: a questionnaire study to quantify and condense reasons for prescribing. *Fam Pract.* **3**:16–20.

Coenen S, Van Royen P, Vermeire E *et al.* (2000). Antibiotics for coughing in general practice: a qualitative decision analysis. *Fam Pract.* **17**:380–5.

Cole NF and O'Connor RW (1987). Estimating current worldwide antibiotic usage: Report of Task Force 1. *Rev Infect Dis.* **9** (Suppl 3): 232–4.

De Maeseneer J (1990). Her voorschrijven van antibioticen vij luchtwegproblemen. Eeen explorened onderzock. *Huisarts Wt.* **33**: 223–6.

De Neeling AJ, Hemms JH and von Klingeren B (1993). Resistentie tegen antibiotica bij routine isolaten van bacteriem in zeven streeklabatoria.

Bilthoven, the Netherlands. Rijksinstitut voor volksge zondheid en milieu-hygeine.

Dosh SA, Hickner JM, Mainous AG 3rd and Ebell MH (2000) Predictors of antibiotic prescribing for non-specific upper respiratory tract infections, acute bronchitis and acute sinusitis. *J Fam Pract.* 49: 407–10.

Finland M (1955) Changing patterns of resistance of certain common pathogenic bacteria to antimicrobial agents. *NEJM.* **252**:570–80.

Friis H, Bro F, Mabeck CE and Vejlsgaard R (1989) Use of antibiotics in general practice in Denmark in 1987. *Scan J Infect Dis* **29**:551–6.

Friis H, Bro F, Eriksen NR *et al.* (1993). The effect of reimbursement on the use of antibiotics. *Scand J Primary Health Care.* 11: 247–51.

Gonzales R, Steiner JF and Sande MA (1997) Antibiotic prescribing for adults with colds, upper respiratory tract infections and bronchitis by ambulatory care physicians. *JAMA.* **278**: 901–4.

Grol R and Wensing M (1999) Patients' expectations with respect to general practice care: an international comparison. *Fam Pract.* 16: 4–11.

Hamm RM, Hicks RJ and Bemden RA (1996). Antibiotics and respiratory infections: are patients more satisfied when expectations are met? *J Fam Pract.* 43: 56–62.

Howie JG and Hutchinson KR (1978). Antibiotics and respiratory illness in general practice: prescribing policy and workload. *BMJ.* **2**:1342.

Hueston WJ, Eberlein C, Johnson D and Mainous AJ (1998). Criteria used by physicians to differentiate sinusitis from viral upper respiratory tract infections. *J Fam Pract.* **46**: 487–92.

Hutchinson JM and Foley RN (1999). Method of physician remuneration and rates of antibiotic prescribing. *CMAJ.* 160: 1013–17.

Hutchinson JM, Jelinsky S, Hefferton D *et al.* (2001). Role of diagnostic labelling in antibiotic prescribing. *Can Fam Physician.* 47: 1217–24.

Institute of Medicine (1989). *Human health risks associated with the sub-therapeutic use of penicillin or tetracycline in animal food.* Washington, DC: National Academy Press, pp. 65–7.

Jackson MA, Shelton S, Nelson JD, McCracken GH (1984). Relatively penicillin-resistant pneumococcal infections in children. *Pediatr Inf Dis J.* **2**: 129–32.

Kellner JD and Ford-Jones EL (1999) Streptococcus pneumoniae carriage in children attending 59 Canadian child care centres. Toronto Child Care Study Group. *Arch Pediatr Adolesc Med.* **153**: 495–502.

Kristinsson KJ (1997). The effect of antimicrobial use and other risk factors on antimicrobial resistance in pneumococci. *Microbiol Drug Resistance.* **3**: 117–23.

Kunin CM (1993). Resistance to antimicrobial drugs: a world-wide calamity. *Ann Intern Med* 118: 557–61.

Mainous AJ, Zoorob RJ, Oler M and Hayned DN (1997) Patients' knowledge of upper respiratory tract infections: implications for antibiotic expectations and unnecessary utilization. *J Fam Pract.* 45: 75–8.

Majeed A and Wrigley T (2002). Antibiotic prescribing rates in England are falling. *BMJ.* **325**: 340.

McCaig LF and Hughes JM (1995) Trends in antimicrobial prescribing among office-based physicians in the US. *JAMA* **278**: 2414–19.

McCaig LF, Besser RE and Hughes RM. (2002) Trends in antimicrobial prescribing rates for children and adolescents. *JAMA* **287**: 3096–102.

Murray S, Del Mar C, O'Rourke P (2000) Predictors of antibiotic prescription for respiratory tract infections: a pilot. *Fam Practice.* **17**: 386–8.

Nasrin D, Collignon PJ, Roberts L *et al.* (2002). Effect of beta lactam antibiotic use in children on pneumococcal resistance to penicillin: prospective cohort study. *BMJ.* **324**: 28–31.

National Ambulatory Medical Care Survey, 1994. http://www.cdc.gov/nchs/about/major/ahcd/namcsdes.htm

National Prescribing Service News(2002) Issue 21 (May), Surrey Hills, Australia 2010.

Nava J, Bella F, Garau J, *et al.* 1994) Predictive factors for invasive disease due to penicillin-resistant *Streptococcus pneumoniae*; a population-based study. *Clin Inf Dis.* **19**: 884–90.

Nowak R. (1994) Hungary sees an improvement in penicillin resistance. *Science.* **264**: 364.

Nyquist AC, Gonzales R, Steiner JF and Sande MA (1998) Antibiotic prescribing for children with colds, URTIs and bronchitis by ambulatory physicians in the United States. *JAMA.* **279**: 875–7.

Pechere JC (2001) Patients' interviews and the misuse of antibiotics. *Clin Infect Dis.* **33** (Supplement 3): 170–3.

Rautakorpi UM, Klaukka T, Honkenen B *et al.* (2001). Antibiotic use by indication: a basis for active antibiotic policy in the community. *Scan J Infect Dis.* **33**: 922–6.

Seppala H, Klaukka T, Vuopi-Varkila J *et al.* (1997). The effects of changes in the consumption of macrolide antibiotics on erythromycin resistance in group A streptococci in Finland. *NEJM.* **337**: 441–6.

Soares S, Kristinsson KJ, Musser JM and Thomasz A (1993) Evidence for the introduction of a multi-resistant clone of serotype 6B *Streptococcus pneumoniae* from Spain to Iceland in the late 1980s. *J Infect Dis.* **168**: 158–63.

Steinman MA, Gonzales R, Linder JA and Landefeld CS (2003) Changing use of antibiotics in community-based out-patient practice, 1991–1999. *Annals Int Med* **138**: 525–33.

Stephenson MJ, Henry N and Norman GR (1988) Factors influencing antibiotic use in acute respiratory tract infections in family practice. *Can Fam Physician.* **34**: 2149–52.

Thomas KB (1978) The consultation and the therapeutic illusion. *BMJ.* **1**: 1327–8.

Turnidge JD, Bell JM and Collignon PJ (1999) Rapidly emerging antimicrobial resistance in *Streptococcus pneumonia* in Australia. *Med J Aust.* **170**: 152–5.

Van Duijn H, Kuyvenhoven M, Jones RT *et al.* (2003) Patients' views on respiratory tract symptoms and antibiotics. *Br J Gen Pract.* **53**: 491–2.

Vinson DC and Lutz LJ (1993) The effect of parental expectations on treatment of children with a cough: report from ASPEN. *J Fam Pract.* **37**: 23–7.

Watson RL, Dowell SF, Jayaraman M *et al.* (1999) Antimicrobial use of paediatric upper respiratory tract infections: reported practice, actual practice and parent beliefs. *Pediatrics.* **104**: 1251–7.

Williams S, Weinmann J, Dale J and Newman S (1995) Patient expectations: what do primary care patients want from their GP and how far does meeting expectations affect patient satisfaction? *Fam Pract.* **12**: 193–201.

Chapter 13

Strategies for promoting change

The general practitioner is like a barmaid in a gin shop, facing overwhelming demand to chemically alter customers' experience of the world.

Dr Marshall Marinker

Change is not made without inconvenience, even from worse to better.
Dr Samuel Johnson

GPs continue to prescribe antibiotics at high rates for conditions whose causes are known to be usually viral or, even if they are possibly bacterial, from which most patients will recover without the use of antibiotics. There are some well-written evidence-based algorithms and clinical decision rules which, if followed, would substantially reduce antibiotic prescribing and costs. Why then do GPs ignore the scientific evidence and persist in what seems at first glance to be an irrational behaviour? To understand this, we need to look at doctors' attitudes to and expectations of their patients and their own work. We shall also look at what patients think, because this also influences what doctors do and prescribe.

Doctors' reasons for prescribing

Some of the earliest research on prescribing for ARIs was conducted by Dr John Howie in Scotland. He mailed illustrated booklets containing photos and information about 16 patients with sore throats to 1000 GPs. A standard medical history was combined with various combinations of social and psychological factors, and GPs were asked whether they would have prescribed antibiotics for each particular patient. It was found that social and psychological factors significantly affected the GPs' prescribing decisions. Increased rates of antibiotic prescribing were associated with factors such as distance from the patient's home to the doctor's surgery, an imminent university examination, an imminent holiday, stress in the mother of a young child, a sibling in hospital with pneumonia, and an imminent job interview. Howie concluded that 'An apparently simple form of management for a physical illness may be substantially influenced by clinical information of a non-physical nature' (Howie, 1976).

Another study by John Howie looked at GP prescribing for new cases of respiratory infection. It was found that GPs spent less time deciding on management than deciding on diagnosis, which suggests that prescribing might be a quicker and less reflective act (Howie and Hutchinson, 1978).

- Doctors have many reasons for prescribing against the clinical evidence. In order of stated frequency, the commonest reasons are as follows:
  - to satisfy patient expectation
  - to satisfy patient demand
  - to preserve the doctor–patient relationship
  - to conform with the doctor's prescribing habit
  - to relieve pressure on time
  - use of antibiotics as a placebo
  - belief that antibiotics are not ineffective
  - diagnostic uncertainty
  - perception that the patient is really sick
  - perception that the patient is at high risk
  - knowledge that antibiotics have worked for this patient before.
- The doctor's perception that the patient wants antibiotics is the strongest factor, but doctors overestimate how many patients expect antibiotics.
- Social and psychological factors are as important as clinical ones in influencing the decision as to whether or not to prescribe antibiotics.
- When doctors prescribe antibiotics diagnostic labelling commonly occurs.

A study by Dr Samuel Coenen in Belgium (Coenen *et al.*, 2000) found that the decision as to whether or not to prescribe an antibiotic was determined more by doctor-related factors (having missed a case of pneumonia in the past, time pressure, fear of losing patients) than by patient-related factors. The more uncertain the GP was about the diagnosis, the more likely it was that antibiotics would be prescribed. The best independent predictor of antibiotic prescribing was the individual doctor's antibiotic prescribing rate (in other words, the habit of the individual GP), followed closely by 'diagnostic labelling.' A study of antibiotic prescriptions written for otitis media by GPs, conducted in the Netherlands by Dr Roger Damoiseaux (Damoiseux *et al.*,1999) in order to determine whether the prescriptions followed the guidelines of the Dutch College of General Practitioners for managing this condition, found that 77% of the prescriptions did not follow the guidelines. The GPs most often gave medical reasons for prescribing – the illness was severe, or the patient had had previous ear problems, was very young or was in a high-risk group.

A study by Kumar *et al.* (2002), which aimed to investigate why GPs in the UK prescribe antibiotics for sore throat, used grounded theory techniques for conducting interviews with 40 GPs. Analysis revealed four dominant themes, namely the benefits of antibiotics to some patients, external pressure to prescribe antibiotics, maintaining the doctor–patient relationship, and feeling comfortable with prescribing.

MacFarlane and colleagues of Nottingham University found that GPs prescribed antibiotics for cough more often for older patients and for those with underlying diseases, discoloured sputum, shortness of breath, wheezing, fever, signs on chest examination and 'other factors.' 'Other factors' included patient pressure, social factors, GP work pressure, and previous experience with the same patient. These researchers concluded that 'The decision concerning the use and choice of antibiotics is a complex interaction between patient, doctor and disease, being affected not only by clinical factors, but also by social and psychological elements; such issues need to be considered when developing relevant guidelines for primary care' (MacFarlane *et al.*, 1997).

In another UK study, by Dr Chris Butler's group in South Wales, GPs were interviewed with a view to better understanding the reasons for antibiotic prescribing for sore throat (Butler *et al.*, 1998). The doctors knew of the evidence for the marginal effectiveness of antibiotics for this condition, yet often prescribed in order to maintain good relationships with patients. Possible patient benefit outweighed the theoretical community risk of development of resistant bacteria. Most doctors felt uncomfortable prescribing 'against the evidence', and realized that it probably increased their workload. Doctors thought that explaining the difference between bacterial and viral infection often confused patients, and they found giving such explanations time-consuming and difficult. Other doctor-related reasons were also given, including habit, a desire to ease the patient, experience of negative events in the past, a desire to ease the doctor, a consultation taking place just before the weekend, or the patient being about to go on holiday.

Several studies have found that doctors feel more confident about making 'tough' prescribing decisions when they know the patient well, but in the increasingly popular walk-in clinics, the doctor is unlikely to know many of the patients whom he or she sees. Even in traditionally organized surgeries, a high proportion of patients with ARIs are otherwise young and healthy, so that perhaps even their own family doctor does not know them very well.

Professor Alvan Feinstein of Yale University School of Medicine (Feinstein, 1985) has postulated a very interesting hypothesis about doctors' prescribing behaviour. He suggests that doctors use a qualitative rather than a quantitative decision model: 'They identify the result that will cause most chagrin, and they avoid the decision option which will lead to it.' For example, the GP looking at a sore throat has to decide whether to treat it immediately, not treat it, or do a test and wait for the results. Individual GPs will choose the option that causes them least chagrin, so they will often prescribe antibiotics straight away.

Patients' attitudes

- Not all patients want an antibiotic prescription for an ARI.
- When given a prescription, not all patients cash it.
- A high proportion of the public believes that antibiotics are an appropriate treatment for coughs, colds and influenza. This group has faith in the power of antibiotics, and expresses satisfaction with high-prescribing GPs.
- Many patients believe that coloured sputum or nasal discharge is a reason to take antibiotics.
- Other patients are sceptical about antibiotics, and consider that they should only be used as a last resort. They prefer to practise self-care when ill, and come to the GP for an accurate diagnosis and reassurance.
- GPs do not appear to be very good at judging patient expectations and attitudes.

Professor Nicky Britten in the UK has done a number of interesting studies on patient attitudes (Britten, 1995; Britten and Okumene, 1997). She found that patients' views about their doctors' prescribing habits ranged from those who wanted more help with their symptoms (who said that doctors under-prescribe) to those who were aware of doctors' pressure of work (who said that GPs over-prescribe). Not all patients wanted a prescription, or cashed it once they had been given one. It was found that two broad sets of attitudes were present in patients who saw their GP. One group had a preference for self-care and the other group had a preference for drug treatment. It was concluded that 'Doctors seemed more aware of the pressure to prescribe than of the preference for self-care'.

An American survey by Dr Robert Hamm (Hamm *et al.*, 1996) of patients with an ARI found that patients were more likely to be satisfied if the doctor explained the illness and they understood the treatment choice, than if they received antibiotics.

In Australia, the National Prescribing Service, a government-funded organisation, used patient focus groups to explore what consumers want when they visit the doctor with an ARI (NPS, 2002). It was found that most participants 'rarely wanted a medicine prescribed for a cold. They wanted to be accurately diagnosed and to be reassured. They wanted to be told to go home and rest, if that was appropriate'. In general, focus group participants thought that antibiotics should be used 'only as a last resort.' Nearly all participants felt that as much information as possible about the side-effects of antibiotics would be desirable, and that insufficient information was currently available. However, 40% of those surveyed thought that an antibiotic was appropriate for coughs, colds and flu.

A survey of 5379 people from nine countries, conducted by Dr Jean Pechere of Geneva (Pechere, 2001), revealed that 87% of respondents thought that antibiotics speed up recovery from infectious diseases, and 74% perceived them as 'strong drugs.' Few individuals believed that antibiotics should be taken for the common cold, but the majority believed that they should be taken for sore throat (72%), fever (67%), earache (65%), thick catarrh (64%), severe cough (65%) and flu (64%). Most patients visiting their doctor with acute respiratory symptoms would expect to receive antibiotics.

In 1997 the World Health Organization reported that European doctors cited patient pressure as the most important reason why they prescribed antibiotics (WHO, 2000). The same report found that in the USA, 95% of physicians surveyed had seen an average of 7 patients in the past 6 months who had requested antibiotics as a result of advertising. In total, 70% of physicians admitted that patient pressure compelled them to prescribe drugs which they might otherwise have avoided using.

Dr John MacFarlane of Nottingham University studied the attitudes of adult patients with ARIs, and found that 90% of patients thought that antibiotics would help, and 87% expected a prescription. Patient pressure commonly caused doctors to prescribe even when they thought that antibiotics were not needed. Indeed, doctors thought that antibiotics were definitely indicated for only 1% of the patients who pressured them. The researchers concluded that 'Patients who consult with acute respiratory symptoms often believe that they need antibiotics, and demand them; this has a significant influence on prescribing, even when the doctor judges that antibiotics are not needed' (MacFarlane *et al.*, 1997).

A prospective study by Mainous *et al.* (1997) of children with cough attending practices in the USA found that when the doctor assessed that there was a parental expectation of antibiotic treatment, the likelihood of a diagnosis of 'bronchitis' being made and an antibiotic being prescribed was doubled. If the doctor thought that the parents did not expect antibiotics, there was an increased likelihood of a diagnosis of 'viral upper respiratory tract infection' rather than 'bronchitis' being made, and an antibiotic was far less likely to be prescribed. Another survey, of adults with ARIs in

Lexington, Kentucky, conducted by the same investigators (Mainous, 1996), found that 72% of respondents would seek care if they had a condition of 5 days' duration with cough, sore throat and discoloured nasal discharge. In total, 79% said that they thought antibiotics would be effective for such a condition. Higher level of education was related to the belief that antibiotics would be more effective for discoloured than for clear discharge. It was concluded that 'Patients lack understanding of the normal presentation of an upper respiratory infection and the effectiveness of antibiotics in treating them; they are also confused about the meaning of a discoloured discharge'.

A Swedish study conducted by Dr Jonas Lundkvist of Uppsala (Lundkvist *et al.*, 2002) found that a high rate of antibiotic prescribing was related to high overall patient satisfaction with the GP consultation. A high frequency of antibiotic prescriptions might reflect a general tendency among GPs to give priority to maintaining a good relationship with patients.

Some patients seem to be only too aware of what influences doctors to prescribe antibiotics. An interesting study in the US (Scott *et al.*, 2001) found that patients were able to exert pressure on their doctor to prescribe, using tactics such as suggesting candidate diagnoses ('It's my bronchitis again, doc') that are more likely to elicit an antibiotic prescription, or exaggerating the severity of their symptoms or their lack of social support.

Although patient demand may be one of the main drivers for unnecessary prescribing, the evidence suggests that the situation is complex, and at least as much stimulus comes from physicians themselves as from patient-related factors. Further evidence for the complex reasons for prescribing will probably only be obtained from qualitative research. We still need to be much more aware of the process of clinical consultations – especially how and how often patients make their expectations known, how doctors assess patient communications, and how well the doctor and patient communicate with each other.

Changing GP behaviour

- Attempts to change GP behaviour by introducing clinical guidelines have usually been unsuccessful.
- Active methods work better than passive ones.
- Multifaceted interventions work better than single ones.
- The following have been found to be almost completely ineffective:
  - medical conferences
  - traditional continuing medical education (CME) lectures

- – mailing guidelines to GPs
- – printing guidelines in journals
- – simple feedback of GP performance
- – complicated recommendations.
- The following are sometimes effective:
  - – academic detailing
  - – small group CME
  - – peer education
  - – simple repeated recommendations
  - – computer reminders (in automated surgeries).

There is a very large literature on methods of changing the behaviour of doctors and other healthcare professionals. The Cochrane Library alone contains seven systematic reviews in this area. An overview of systematic reviews of professional behaviour change interventions, by Dr Jeremy Grimshaw and colleagues (Grimshaw *et al.*, 2001), found no fewer than 41 reviews. A wide range of interventions had been tested. In general, passive interventions were ineffective and unlikely to result in behaviour change. Most other interventions were effective under some circumstances, but none were effective under all circumstances. Promising approaches to changing doctors' prescribing behaviour included educational outreach and automatic reminders. Multifaceted interventions that targeted different barriers to change were more likely to be effective than single interventions. This review concluded that 'When people are planning changes they often adopt a naive and opportunistic attitude. A strategy is usually quickly chosen and does not have the expected result. Until we have a better understanding, the most practical advice to individuals responsible for changing and improving practice is to be aware of their own assumptions about human behaviour and change. There are many approaches to changing clinical care for patients and implementing guidelines, all of which have some value, depending on the changes aimed for, the target group, the clinical setting, and the barriers and facilitators found there'.

Continuing medical education

Formal continuing medical education (CME) conferences and the distribution of printed materials have little effect on doctors' behaviour unless they are reinforced by other strategies. Many studies have shown that education at an individual or small group level and peer education are more effective strategies for changing doctors' antibiotic-prescribing behaviour. Establishing credibility, defining clear objectives for behaviour change, and repetition and reinforcement are all-important for peer education.

A review by Dr Jonathan Lomas (Lomas, 1991) of studies of passive dissemination of consensus-derived recommendations concluded that there was little evidence that such dissemination alone resulted in behaviour change. Another review by Dr Robert Grilli (Grilli and Lomas, 1994), which assessed studies of factors associated with guideline compliance by doctors, found that compliance was lower for recommendations that were more complex and less easy to pilot.

Educational outreach

A systematic review by Dr Stephen Soumerai at Harvard Medical School (Soumerai and Avorn, 1990) examined studies of educational outreach to doctors. All of the interventions consisted of several components, including written material and conferences, reminders and audit. The review concluded that 'Educational outreach visits, particularly when combined with social marketing, appear to be a promising approach to modifying health professionals' behaviour, especially prescribing'. Another systematic review looked at the effect of CME. There was substantial variation in the complexity of targeted behaviours, and substantial heterogeneity in the results. The reviewers concluded that 'Interactive workshops can result in moderate changes in professional practice. Didactic sessions alone are unlikely to change professional practice' (Davis *et al.*, 1995).

Feedback

Providing feedback to doctors about their own antibiotic-prescribing behaviour has been a successful technique for achieving change behaviour. Feedback may be most effective when the system is developed with local input, and when clinicians accept that the measures are important, fair and relevant to their own practices. New communication technologies such as the internet enhance the potential to disseminate guidelines and to provide feedback. Computer-assisted decision support systems have been used effectively to support antibiotic prescribing in hospitals, but to date there have been no general practice studies of this approach.

Educating opinion leaders

One limitation of all intervention strategies is that some providers will participate and others will not. Convincing local opinion leaders to change their own practices will result in eventual diffusion of change. For this reason, identifying and educating opinion leaders as a priority group may be effective, particularly if resources are limited. Educating future healthcare providers (nurses, doctors and pharmacists in training) may also have a long-term impact, and is a useful strategy if focused on current providers.

Multi-faceted strategies

Following their experience of several intervention trials in the USA, Belongia *et al.* (2001) suggested an ideal but very expensive approach:

> A multifaceted approach is needed to increase the public's understanding of antibiotic resistance and to change expectations about use of antibiotics. The key elements should include a public education campaign, clinic-based education, and community outreach activities. Conducting a public relations campaign with paid advertising is an effective but expensive strategy to change health-related behaviour. Educating the public about the difference between bacterial and viral infections, and the potential risks of taking antibiotics, is more complex than other health education messages because the risk to benefit ratio is less clear. Educational interventions for patients and their parents at outpatient clinics must be an important part of any public education campaign. Information provided during a medical consultation is immediately relevant and is likely to be authoritative. Clinicians should distribute educational materials designed for patients. Medical providers should also seek opportunities for community partnerships to disseminate such messages widely. Interventions should be supported by national and local policies that promote judicious antibiotic use. National goals to reduce unnecessary use should be set. Progress towards these goals should be monitored. Databases should be established to support feedback interventions and programme evaluation.

A detailed *Effective Health Care* bulletin from the Centre for Reviews and Dissemination at the University of York concluded that guidelines can change clinical practice, and were more likely to be effective if they took account of local circumstances, were disseminated by an active educational intervention, and were implemented using patient-specific reminders (University of York, 1994). There was inconclusive evidence as to whether guidelines that had been developed locally were more likely to be effective than those developed nationally.

Educational theories of changing behaviour

Educational theorists have used various models of change to improve understanding of the behaviour of healthcare professionals and to guide the development and implementation of interventions intended to change behaviour. Learning theory offers an explanation of how behaviour is changed and maintained. Social cognition models regard factors such as beliefs, attitudes and intentions as central influences in shaping behaviour.

In particular three sets of beliefs have emerged as important in determining behaviour:

1 perceived benefits weighed against perceived barriers
2 perceptions about the attitudes of important others
3 belief in one's own abilities.

Models also describe how individuals pass through a sequence of stages of change. The commonest stage model postulates that five stages occur, namely pre-contemplation, contemplation, preparation, action, and maintenance of the change. Another approach, postulated by Rogers (1983), suggests that people can be divided into innovators, early adopters, part of the early majority, part of the late majority, and laggards.

If change does occur in a sequence of stages, and different doctors are at different stages, it is clear that a variety of techniques will be needed to secure change, as groups differ in their needs and the degree to which they are prepared to change. Change models suggest that individuals and organisations differ in their receptivity to change, and perceive different barriers and benefits to change. Barriers to change can be formidable, but implementation programmes can be successful if they use interventions and activities that reduce restraining forces, such as increased workload, lack of time, poor communication, traditional working practices, and individual and organisational resistance to change.

Although a group of doctors may agree in theory to change its behaviour, the survey conducted by Dr Damoiseaux (Damoiseaux *et al.*, 1999) in the Netherlands found that a doctor faced with an individual patient would tend to err on the side of caution or rely on 'personal experience' rather than research-based evidence. In the UK, a Framework for Appropriate Care Throughout Sheffield (Eve *et al*, 1997) programme found that getting agreement on whether a topic is even worth tackling depends on the following factors.

1 The issue must be perceived as a significant problem.
2 The proposed change must follow national policy.
3 The problems can be solved by change.
4 There is no strong opposition to change from key individuals.
5 The change must not consume too many resources.
6 There must not be a gap between what doctors say publicly they are prepared to do and what they are actually prepared to do.

Finally, we must not forget that there is a natural tendency to return to previous practice patterns, unless there is constant motivation together with reminders to change.

- Interventions that have been used, in various combinations, include the following:
  - provider education (printed materials, small group and academic detailing)
  - patient education (printed materials and discussion groups)
  - community education (printed and electronic media)
  - practice profiling and feedback.
- Such multifaceted interventions have been used in several major trials in the USA. They are very expensive to mount and difficult to maintain.
- Individual GP practices have used the following:
  - verbal advice and leaflets
  - practice education and leaflets.

Provider education

In New South Wales, a two-step educational intervention trial conducted by Dr Nicholas Zwar (Zwar *et al.*, 1999), which provided education and then feedback of behaviour to GP trainees, reduced antibiotic prescribing for ARIs from 25% to 20%, compared with an increase from 25% to 32% in the control group. Five years later, members of the intervention group were found to have maintained their changed behaviour and, interestingly, the prescribing rates in the control group had decreased during that period, so that there was no longer a significant difference in behaviour between the two groups. Also in Australia, a trial was conducted by Dr Georgio de Santis (de Santis *et al.*, 1994), using an educational tool for tonsillitis followed by academic detailing of GPs by a pharmacist. In the intervention group, appropriate antibiotic use increased from 61% to 88%, compared with an increase from 53% to 72% in the control group.

Individual interventions

General practices in Norway took part in a trial conducted by Dr Signe Flottorp (Flottorp *et al.*, 2002) of tailored interventions to improve the management of sore throat. Patients were given educational material, GPs were given decision support and therapeutic reminders from computers, GPs received an increase in their fee for telephone consultations, and the GPs and their practice assistants attended interactive case-based educational sessions. After this expensive intervention, patients with sore throat were only 3% less likely to be prescribed antibiotics. Also in Norway, a trial by Dr Fagan (Fagan, 2001) found that an educational intervention for general practices reduced the antibiotic-prescribing rate for acute bronchitis from 87% to 71% (interestingly, the rate of antibiotic pre-scribing for 'bronchitis' was reduced, but more cases of 'pneumonia' were diagnosed).

In the USA, Dr Ralph Gonzales (Gonzales *et al.*, 1999) conducted a non-randomised trial of patient education combined with clinician education, practice profiling and academic detailing. At the full intervention sites in Denver, Colorado, four primary care practices used an intervention consisting of household and surgery-based patient educational materials, as well as a clinician intervention consisting of education, practice profiling and academic detailing. At these sites, antibiotic prescribing for acute bronchitis in adults decreased from 74% to 48%; in the control sites, antibiotic prescribing was not reduced.

Also in the USA, Belongia *et al.* (2001) asked primary care physicians in northern Wisconsin who provided paediatric care to take part in a non-randomised community intervention trial. Clinic staff received printed educational materials and small-group presentations, and printed material was distributed to parents through clinics, childcare facilities and commu-nity organisations. The median number of antibiotic prescriptions decreased by 19% in the intervention group compared with 8% in the control region.

One of the most intensive multifaceted trials was conducted in Knox County, Tennessee, by Dr John Perz and colleagues (Perz *et al.*, 2002). Provider education consisted of lectures to 150 key providers, presenta-tions at many hospital staff meetings, and the distribution of new pre-scribing guidelines and related articles in a newsletter to all 1500 physicians in the area. Parent education consisted of the distribution of pamphlets to parents of all children in K-grade 3, the distribution of patient education materials to 250 key providers, provision of pamphlets to parents of every newborn baby, and public education (distribution of 30 000 pamphlets, communication through television, radio and newspapers, and distribution of pamphlets to flu-vaccine recipients and all community pharmacies). There was a 19% decrease in the intervention group, compared with a 5% decrease in the control group.

In Nottingham in the UK, Dr John MacFarlane conducted a trial to determine whether verbal advice plus an information leaflet describing the uncertain value of antibiotics would reduce antibiotic use more than verbal advice given alone for adults with acute bronchitis (Macfarlane *et al.*, 2002). Fewer patients in the intervention group took their antibiotics (47% vs. 62%). The groups did not differ in their re-consultation rates after 4 weeks (11% vs. 13%). Also in the UK, one general practice consisting of 14 000 patients in semi-rural Hampshire developed its own evidence-based protocol (Cox *et al.*, 2001) through a feedback and small-group educational process. Once the group had taken the decision to implement this, antibiotic prescriptions for ARIs decreased from 56% to

19%. In Canada, Dr Warren McIsaac and colleagues (McIsaac *et al.*, 1998) used an information package on throat infections for GPs, plus a sore throat scorecard and a recording form for use during consultations for sore throat, to see whether these interventions affected GPs' antibiotic-prescribing rates. There was an overall trend towards a reduction in antibiotic prescribing (21%) in physicians who used the intervention package, but a greater reduction (45%) was observed for patients in whom the probability of infection with GABHS was low according to the sore throat decision rule. They concluded that 'Sore throat rules may reduce unnecessary antibiotic prescriptions if physicians are specifically cued to use them during clinical encounters'.

- The most consistently successful method has been delayed prescribing of antibiotics.
- Other methods that have sometimes worked, but usually only to a small degree, include the following:
  - increased consultation length/discussion time
  - unanimous practice policy decision
  - practice profiling/feedback
  - interactive workshops for small groups of GPs
  - use of nurse practitioners rather than GPs
  - academic detailing by fellow GPs.

Delayed prescriptions

The 'delayed prescription' is a useful management tool for the GP who feels uncomfortable not prescribing antibiotics. By asking the patient to wait for a few days and to use the prescription only if they are not getting better a power struggle is avoided, and patients participate in their own management. Delayed prescribing has not only decreased antibiotic use, but has also changed patients' perceptions about respiratory illnesses and decreased subsequent visits for uncomplicated respiratory illness. Dr Paul Little's group in southern England found that giving adults who had sore throat, or children with otitis media, a delayed prescription (to be used, if needed, after 3 days) did not affect outcomes (Little *et al.*, 1997, 2001). In Auckland, New Zealand, Arroll found that if a delayed prescription was given to adult patients who presented with common cold symptoms and requested an antibiotic, far fewer people took the antibiotic, and outcomes did not differ (Arroll *et al.* 2002). In the USA, a similar study by Dr Glen Couchman showed that although 96% of patients were satisfied because they had received the delayed prescription, only 50% actually cashed it, and the overall prescribing rate was reduced by 31% (Couchman *et al.*,

2000). In Scotland, an open randomised trial of delayed prescribing of antibiotics for patients with cough was conducted by Dr Jon Dowell, and it was found that over 50% of the delayed prescriptions were not cashed (Dowell *et al.*, 2001).

Nurse practitioners

Some doctors ask a nurse practitioner to see all patients with ARIs. The effect seems to vary according to the setting and the training of the nurse. In Wales, a study by Dr Butler's group found that the nurse practitioner prescribed antibiotics for a much smaller proportion of patients (Butler *et al.*, 2001). In the year following the visit to the nurse, the patients consulted less often and received antibiotics for ARIs less often than in the year preceding the visit. On the other hand, a study in the USA by Dr Steven Dosh (Dosh *et al.*, 2000) found that nurse practitioners were four times more likely to prescribe antibiotics than doctors.

A single physician or a group of doctors can unilaterally decide to change their own behaviour. In 1997, a group of English GPs decided to change their policy with regard to the routine use of antibiotics for children with otitis media. Over a period of 12 months, the median number of pre-scriptions in the practice decreased from 75 to 47 per month, and the number of amoxycillin prescriptions decreased by one-third (Cates, 1999).

It seems clear that there is no single simple and easy way to change GPs' antibiotic-prescribing habits. The most successful interventions have used several techniques simultaneously, targeting both doctors and patients. Doctors already know about the limited efficacy of these drugs. They need to be more aware of their non-medical motives for prescribing antibiotics, and how to determine which patients are looking for advice and reassur-ance, rather than for medication.

References

Arroll B, Keneally T and Kerse B (2002) Do delayed prescriptions reduce the consumption of antibiotics for the common cold? A single-blind controlled trial. *J Fam Pract.* **51**: 337–8.

Belongia EA, Sullivan BJ, Chyou PH, Madagame E, Reed KE and Schwartz B (2001) A community *intervention* trial to promote judicious antibiotic use and reduce penicillin-resistant *Streptococcus pneumoniae* carriage in children. *Pediatrics.* **108**: 575–83.

Britten N (1995) Patients' demand for prescriptions in primary care. *BMJ.* **310**: 1084–5.

Britten N, Okumenne O (1997) The influence of patients' hopes of receiving a prescription on doctors' perceptions and the decision to prescribe. *BMJ.* **315**: 1506–10.

Butler CC, Rollnick S, Pill R *et al.* (1998) Understanding the culture of prescribing:

qualitative study of general practitioners' and patients' perceptions of anti-biotics for sore throats. *BMJ.* **317**: 637–42.

Butler CC, Kinnersley P, Prout H *et al.* (2001) Antibiotics and shared decision making in primary care. *J Antimicrob Chemother.* **48**: 435–40

Cates C (1999). An evidence-based approach to reducing antibiotic use in children with acute otitis media; controlled before-and-after study. *BMJ.* **318**: 715–16.

Coenen S, van Royen P, Vermeire E *et al.* (2000) Antibiotics for coughing in general practice: a qualitative decision study. *Fam Practice.* **17**: 382–5.

Couchman GR, Roscoe TJ and Forjuoh GN (2000) Back-up prescriptions for common respiratory symptoms; patient satisfaction and fill rates. *J Fam Pract.* **49**: 907–13.

Cox CM and Jones M (2001) Is it possible to decrease antibiotic prescribing in primary care? An analysis of outcomes in the management of patients with sore throats. *Fam Pract.* **18**: 9–13.

Damoiseaux RA, de Melker RA, Ausems MJ and van Balen FA (1999) Reasons for non guideline-based antibiotic prescriptions in the Netherlands. *Fam Pract.* **16**: 50–3.

Davis DA, Thompson MA, Oxman A and Haynes RB (1995) Changing physicians' performance: a systematic review of the effects of continuing medical education strategies. *JAMA.* **274**: 700–5.

de Santis G, Harvey KJ, Howard D and Mashford ML (1994) Improving the quality of antibiotic prescribing patterns in general practice: the role of educational intervention. *Med J Aust.* **160**: 502–5.

Dosh SA, Hickner J, Mainous AG and Ebell MH (2000) Predictors of antibiotic prescribing for non-specific upper respiratory tract infections, a cute sinusitis and acute bronchitis. *J Fam Pract.* **49**: 407–10.

Dowell J, Pitkethly M, Bain J and Martin S (2001) A randomized controlled trial of delayed prescribing as a strategy for managing uncomplicated respiratory tract infections in primary care. *Br J Gen Pract.* **51**: 200–5.

Eve R, Golton I and Hodgkin P (1997) *Learning from FACTS: Lessons from the Framework for Appropriate Health Care throughout Sheffield project.* Sheffield University, Sheffield.

Fagan MS (2001) Can use of antibiotics in acute bronchitis be reduced? *Tiddskr Nor Laegeforen.* **121**: 455–8.

Feinstein A (1985) The 'chagrin' factor and qualitative decision analysis. *Arch Int Medicine.* **145**: 1257–9.

Flottorp S, Oxman AD, Havelstrud K and Herrin J (2002) Cluster-randomized controlled trial of tailored interventions to improve the management of urinary tract infections in women and sore throat. *BMJ.* **325**: 367–8.

Gonzales R, Steiner J, Lum A and Barrett PH (1999) Decreasing antibiotic use in ambulatory practice: impact of a multi-dimensional intervention on the treatment of uncomplicated acute bronchitis in adults. *JAMA.* **281**: 1512–19.

Grilli R and Lomas J (1994) Evaluating the message: the relationship between compliance rate and the subject of a practice guideline. *Med Care.* **32**: 202–3.

Grimshaw J, Shirran L, Thomas R and Mowat G (2001) Changing provider behaviour: an overview of systematic reviews of interventions. *Med Care.* **39**: 112–45.

Hamm RM, Hicks RJ and Bemden RA (1996) Antibiotics and respiratory infections: are patient more satisfied when expectations are met? *J Fam Pract.* **43**: 56–62.

Howie JGR (1976) Clinical judgment and antibiotic use in general practice. *BMJ.* 2: 1061–4.

Howie JGR and Hutchinson KR (1978) Antibiotics and respiratory illness in general practice: prescribing policy and workload. *BMJ.* 2: 1342.

Kumar S, Little P and Britten N (2002) Why do general practitioners prescribe antibiotics for sore throat? Grounded theory interview study. *BMJ.* 326: 138.

Little P, Williamson I, Warner G, Gould C, Gantley M and Kinmonth AL (1997). Open randomised trial of prescribing strategies in managing sore throat. *BMJ.* 314: 722–7.

Little P, Gould C, Williamson I, Moore M, Warner G and Dunleavey J (2001) Pragmatic randomised controlled trial of two prescribing strategies for child-hood acute otitis media. *BMJ.* 322: 336–42.

Lomas J (1991) Words without action? The production, dissemination and impact of consensus recommendations. *Ann Rev Pub Health.* 12: 41–65.

Lundkvist J, Akerland I, Borgquist L and Molstadt S (2002) The more time spent on listening, the less time spent on prescribing antibiotics in general practice. *Fam Pract.* 19: 638–40.

MacFarlane J, Holmes W, Macfarlane R and Britten N (1997) Influence of patients' expectations on antibiotic management of acute lower respiratory tract infection in general practice: questionnaire study. *BMJ.* 315: 1211–14.

MacFarlane J, Holmes W, Gard P, Thornhill D (2002) Verbal advice plus an information leaflet reduced antibiotic use in acute bronchitis. *BMJ.* 324: 91–4.

McIsaac WJ and Goel V (1998) Effect of an explicit decision support tool on the decision to prescribe antibiotics for sore throat. *Med Decision Making.* 18: 220–8.

Mainous AG, Hueston WJ and Clark J (1996) Antibiotics and upper respiratory infections: do some folks think there is a cure for the common cold? *J Fam Pract.* 42: 357–61.

Mainous AG III, Zoorob RJ, Oler MJ and Haynes DM (1997) Patient knowledge of upper respiratory infections: implications for antibiotic expectations and unnecessary utilization. *J Fam Pract.* 45: 75–83.

National Prescribing Service News 2002, issue 21. NPS Surrey Hills, NSW Australia 2010.

Pechere JC (2001) Patients' interviews and the misuse of antibiotics. *Clin Infect Dis.* 33 (Supplement 3): 170–3.

Perz JF, Craig AS, Coffey CS and Jorgensen DM (2002) Changes in antibiotic prescribing for children after a community-wide campaign. *JAMA.* 287: 3103–9.

Rogers E (1983) *Diffusions of Innovations.* Free Press, New York.

Scott JG, Cohen D, DiCicco-Bloom B *et al.* (2001) Antibiotic use in acute respiratory infections and the ways patients pressure physicians for a pre-scription. *J Fam Pract.* 50: 853–8.

Soumerai S and Avorn J (1990) Principles of educational outreach to improve clinical decision making. *JAMA.* 263: 548–56.

University of York (1994) *Implementing Clinical Guidelines: can guidelines be used to improve clinical practice?* Effective Health Care bulletin. Centre for Reviews and Dissemination, University of York.

World Health Organization (2000) *Report on Infectious Diseases: overcoming anti-microbial resistance.*WHO, Geneva. www.who.int/infectious-diseases-report/2000

Zwar N, Wolk J, Gordon J and Kehoe L (1999) Influencing antibiotic prescribing in general practice: a trial of prescriber feedback and management guidelines. *Fam Pract.* 16: 1512–19.

Index

absenteeism rates 8
   bronchitis 58
   common colds 15
acoustic reflectometry 40–1, 106–7
acute bronchitis 58–65
   causative agents 12–13, 58–9
   clinical course and diagnosis 58–61, 107
   epidemiology 58–9
   terminology 65
   treatments 61–5
acute otitis media (AOM) 37–47
   causative agents 12–13, 37–8
   clinical course 38–9
   diagnosis and detection 38–41, 106–7
   effusion 45
   other countries 46–7
   prophylaxis 46
   treatments 41–5
acute pneumonia 60, 63
acute respiratory tract infections (ARIs)
   aetiology 11–13
   classification 4
   diagnostic issues 102–9, 118–19
   epidemiology 7–10, 8, 10
   frequency distributions 10
   literature 2–4
   prescribing patterns 111–20
   tests and investigations 103–9
   workload implications 2–3, 9–10
acute rheumatic fever (ARF) 31
acute sinusitis 49–57
   causative agents 12–13, 49–50
   clinical course 50–2
   diagnosis and tests 50–2, 107–8, 118
   epidemiology 49–50
   terminology and prescribing 118
   treatments 52–6
acute sore throat 24–34
   causative agents 13, 24–5
   clinical course 25–6
   clinical decision rules 106, 135
   diagnosis and detection 25–9, 103, 106
   epidemiology 24–5
   treatments 26, 28, 29–34
adrenaline 82, 87

aetiological issues (ARIs) 11–13
   general causative agents 13
amantidine 70, 77
amoxycillin 43–4
antibiotics
   acute bronchitis 61–3
   acute otitis media 41–4
   acute sore throats 28–33
   acute sinusitis 53–6
   bronchiolitis 97
   common colds 17, 20–1
   croup 84
   influenza 70
   patient attitudes 116–19, 126–9
   practitioner attitudes 123–6
   prescribing patterns 111–20
   resistance rates 113–14
   training and education 128–35
   use in food chain 112
   use in other countries 46–7, 61–3,
      114–17, 119–20
anticholinergic drugs 18, 95–6
antigen tests
   acute sore throats 27–8, 106
   bronchiolitis 92, 109
   influenza 69–70
antigenic shift 68
antihistamines
   common cold 18
   sinusitis 53
   antipyretics, common colds 19
antitussives 18, 64–5, 84
antiviral agents
   common cold 16, 20
   influenza prevention 76–7
   influenza treatment 70–1
apnoea, and bronchiolitis 93
ARIs see acute respiratory tract infections
      (ARIs)
Arroll, B and Kenealy, T 20–1
asthma
   and acute bronchitis 61
   and bronchiolitis 91
   and influenza vaccines 75–6
Ausejo, M et al. 85

bacterial meningitis 30–1
beliefs and prescribing 132
Belongia, EA *et al.* 131, 134
beta-agonists 64, 95–7
Bhattacharyya, T *et al.* 107
Bjornson, C *et al.* 86
Boivin, G *et al.* 108
Bordetella pertussis 63
Bordley, C *et al.* 92
breast feeding, and immunity 98–9
Bridges-Webb, C 7–8, 11–12
Britten, N 126
Britten, N and Ukoumunne, O 117
bronchiolitis 90–9
   causative agents 13, 91
   diagnosis 91–3, 109
   epidemiology 90–1
   prophylaxis 98–9
   subsequent wheezing 96–7
   treatments 93–8
bronchodilators 64, 94–5
budenoside 87
Butler, CC *et al.* 116–17, 119, 125, 136

Carman, WF *et al.* 69–70
carrier status 25, 104–5
Cars, O *et al.* 115
Cates, CJ *et al.* 76
Centor, RM 27
change mechanisms 131–3
'chest colds' 65
chest X-rays 104
Christakis, DA *et al.* 93
clinical decision rules 103, 105
   acute sore throats 106, 135
   influenza 108
   use of computer-assisted support
      systems 130
clinical guidelines 128–30
COAD, and influenza vaccines 75–6
codeine 18
Coenen, S *et al.* 116, 117–18, 124
common cold
   causative agents 13, 15–16
   clinical course and diagnosis 16–17, 106
   complications 17
   epidemiology 15–16
   incidence 15
   prevention 21–2
   treatments 17–21
Common Cold Unit (CCU) (Salisbury)
   15–16

*Common Diseases: Their Nature, Incidence and
   Care* (Fry) 2
computer-assisted decision support
   systems 130
continuing medical education (CME)
   129–30
coronaviruses 16
corticosteroids
   and bronchiolitis 96–7
   and croup 84–7, 87–8
Couchman, GR *et al.* 135–6
cough medicines 64–5
   and croup 84
Crombie, DL *et al.* 102–3
croup 80–8
   causative agents 12–13, 81
   clinical course 81–2
   diagnosis 82–3, 109
   epidemiology 80–1
   supportive measures 83–4
   treatments 84–8
CT scans, acute sinusitis 52, 107–8

Damoiseaux, RA *et al.* 42, 124–5, 132
de Bock, GH *et al.* 55
de Maeseneer, J 118
de Melker, RA 3–4
de Santis, G *et al.* 133
decongestants
   cold symptoms 18
   sinusitis 53
Del Mar, CB *et al.* 30
delayed prescriptions 135–6
Denny, FW *et al.* 31
dexamethasone 84–6, 97
dextromorphan 18
diabetes, and vaccine efficacy 75
diagnostic labelling 118
Dosh, SA *et al.* 136
Douglas, RM *et al.* 16

ear infections *see* acute otitis media (AOM)
Eby, GA *et al.* 19
Echinacea
   as prophylactic measure 19
   as treatment 17, 19
educational outreach 130
emergency departments, ARI visits 9–10,
   10
epidemiological studies 7–10, *8, 10*
   common cold 15–16
epinephrine 82, 87, 95
erythromycin resistance 112, 114

Evans, AS 12–13
Everard, ML *et al.* 95–6
expectorants 18

Fagan, MS 133–4
Family Medicine: Principles and Practice
    (Taylor) 3
'fee-for-service' prescribing 117
feedback on prescribing 130
Feinstein, A 125–6
Flores, G and Horwitz, RI 95
Flottorp, S. *et al.* 133
'Framework for Appropriate Care
    Throughout Sheffield' (Eve *et al.*) 132
Friis, H *et al.* 115, 117
Froom, J *et al.* 47
Fry, J 2, 7, *8*, 15

GABHS (Group A beta-haemolytic
    streptococcus) 24–5, 27–33
    see also acute sore throat
Garrison, M *et al.* 96
ginseng, cold prevention studies 22
Glasziou, PP *et al.* 43
glomerulonephritis 31
glucocorticoids 84–7
Goebel, L *et al.* 97
Gonzales, R *et al.* 134
Griffin, S *et al.* 87
Grilli, R and Lomas, J 130
Grimshaw, J *et al.* 129
Gwaltney, J 16

haemagglutinin 68
Haemophilus influenzae 113–14
Hak, E *et al.* 75
Hamm, RM *et al.* 119, 126
Hansen, JG *et al.* 11
Hartling, L *et al.* 95
helium administration 84
Hodgkin, K 2, 7, 80
Honkanen, PO *et al.* 104
hospitalisation, bronchiolitis 90–4, 99
Howie, JG 124
Howie, JG and Hutchinson, KR 21, 102,
    115
Hueston, WJ *et al.* 12
Hutchinson, JM *et al.* 102, 115–16, 117,
    118

imaging studies 52, 104, 107–8
immunoglobulins, and bronchiolitis 97–9
Infectious Diseases Society of America 29

influenza 67–77
    causative agents 13, 68
    clinical course and diagnosis 68–70, 108
    epidemiology 67–8
    pandemic strategies 77
    prevention 71–7
    treatments 70–1
information packages, practitioner/patient
    trials 133–5
interferon 16, 20
ipratropium 18, 95–6
Irwin, RS and Curley, FS 64

Johnson, Dr Samuel 123

Kairys, SW *et al.* 85
Karma, PH *et al.* 39–40
Kellner, JD *et al.* 95, 113
King, DE *et al.* 63
Klassen, TP *et al.* 94
Kolmus, HJ *et al.* 104
Kumar, S *et al.* 125
Kunin, CM 113

learning theories 131–3
Lieberman, D *et al.* 102
Lindbaek, M *et al.* 107–8
Linder, JA and Sim, I 63
literature on ARIs 2–4
Little, P *et al.* 33, 43
Lomas, J 129–30
Low, DE *et al.* 54–5
Luks, D and Anderson, MR 18
Lundkvist, J *et al.* 128
lung disease, and influenza vaccines 75–6

M2 ion-channel blockers 70, 76–7
McConnaichie, KM 91
MacFarlane, J *et al.* 125, 127, 134
McIsaac, WJ *et al.* 135
McWhinney, IR 3
Mainous, AJ *et al.* 127–8
Marcy, M *et al.* 42
Marinker, Dr Marshall 123
Matheson, NJ *et al.* 76–7
meningitis, bacterial 30–1
microbiological tests 103–9
    acute bronchitis 59, 107
    acute sinusitis 51, 107–8
    acute sore throats 27–8, 106
    bronchiolitis 92, 109
    influenza 69–70, 103, 108-
    in-house testing 103–4

monoclonal RSV antibody
  prophylaxis 99
  treatment 98
Monto, AS *et al.* 108
Moraxella catarrhalis 114
Murray, S *et al.* 117
Mycoplasma-associated bronchitis 63
myringotomy 40–1

NAIs (neuraminidase inhibitors) 71, 76–7
nasal discharge 17, 21
Nasrin, D *et al.* 112, 116
National Ambulatory Care Survey
    (NAMCS 1992) 115
Nava, J *et al.* 113
'near-patient' testing 103–4
nebulised adrenaline 82, 87
nebulised steroids 86–7
Netherlands 114
Neto, GM *et al.* 83
neuraminidase inhibitors (NAIs) 71, 76–7
NSAIDs
    acute sore throats 34
    common cold 19
nurse practitioners 136
Nyquist, AC *et al.* 112, 115

OME (otitis media with effusion) 45
  see also acute otitis media (AOM)
oseltamivir 71, 76–7
Osler, Sir William 4, 24, 102
otitis media with effusion (OME) 45
  see also acute otitis media (AOM)
otoscopy 40, 104, 106–7
oxygen administration 84

palivizumab 98, 99
pandemic influenza surveillance 77
parainfluenza viruses
    and bronchiolitis 91–2
    and croup 81
Parker, R *et al.* 85–6
Patel, H *et al.* 96
patient attitudes, to antibiotics 116–19,
    126–9
patient information 133–5
patient satisfaction studies 119
Pauling, Dr Linus 19
PCR (polymerase chain reaction) tests
    69–70
Pechere, JC 127
penicillin
  for acute sore throats 32–3

early clinical trials 31
  resistance patterns 111–14
Perz, JF *et al.* 134
PICNIC (Pediatric Investigators
    Collaborative Network on Infections
    in Canada) 92–3, 94
pneumatic otoscopy 40, 104, 106–7
pneumococcal vaccines, acute otitis media
    prophylaxis 46
polymerase chain reaction (PCR) tests
    69–70
prednisolone 97
prescribing antibiotics
    general patterns 111–20
    patient 'demands' 116–19, 126–9
    practitioner attitudes 123–6
    re-educating practitioners/patients
    128–35
    role of fees and payments 117
    role of nurse practitioners 136
    use of 'delayed prescriptions' 135–6
    see also antibiotics
prophylactic measures
    and antibiotic resistance 112
    acute otitis media 46
    bronchiolitis 98–9
    common cold 16, 21–?
    influenza 71–7
provider education 133
purulence 21

RADTs (rapid antigen detection tests)
    27–8, 69–70, 92, 104, 106
Rakel, RE 3
Randolph, AG and Wang, EEL 97–8
rapid antigen detection tests (RADTs)
    27–8, 69–70, 92, 104, 106
respiratory disease, and influenza vaccines
    75–6
respiratory failure
    bronchiolitis 90–2
    croup 82–3
respiratory syncytial virus (RSV) 91–2
  see also bronchiolitis
rheumatic carditis 31
rheumatic fever 31
rhinoviruses 16
ribavirin 97–9
rimantidine 70, 76–7
Rogers, E 132
Rosenthal, RM 39
RSV (respiratory syncytial virus) 91–2
  see also bronchiolitis

RSV immunoglobulin
  prophylaxis 99
  treatment 98

salbutamol 94–5
Schroeder, K and Fahey, T 18
'self-care' patients 126
sinus puncture 50
smoking, and bronchitis 63
Smucny, J *et al.* 62
SNOT (Sino-Nasal Outcome Test) 107
sore throat decision rules 106, 135
Soumerai, S and Avorn, J 130
sputum colour 21, 60, 117
Staphylococcus aureus 111–12
Steiner, WPR 94
Stephenson, MJ *et al.* 115
steroids
  and bronchiolitis 96–7
  and croup 86–7, 87–8
Straetemans, M *et al.* 46
streptococcal infections, acute sore throat
  24–5, 27–33
Streptococcus pneumoniae 112–13, 114
Streptococcus pyogenes 113–14
stridor 82
Super, DM *et al.* 84–5

Tan, A *et al.* 75
Taverner, D *et al.* 18
Taylor, B *et al.* 21
Taylor, RB 3
tests and investigations *see* imaging studies;
  microbiological tests; viral tests
tetracycline resistance 112
A Textbook of Family Medicine (McWhinney)
  3
Textbook of Family Medicine (Rakel) 3
Thomas, KB 117
TM (tympanic membrane) signs 39–40
tonsillectomies 34
'tonsillitis', diagnosis issues 102
Towards Earlier Diagnosis in General Practice
  (Hodgkin) 2
Turnidge, JD *et al* 113

tympanometry 40, 104, 106–7
Tyrell, DAJ *et al.* 15–16

ultrasonography studies, acute sinusitis 52
University of Adelaide 16
University of Virginia School of Medicine
  16
University of York 131
USA healthcare 9, 115, 117, 119–20

vaccines
  bronchiolitis 99
  common cold 22
  influenza 71–6
  non-compliance 74
  side effects 73
van Bevr, HP *et al.* 81
van Buchem, FL *et al.* 41
van Elden, L *et al.* 69
van Essen, GA *et al.* 74
van Woensel, J and Kinpen, J 94
vapour inhalations 20
Vinson, DC and Lutz, LJ 116, 118
viral tests, influenza 103, 108
vitamin C
  as prophylactic measure 19
  as treatment 17, 19

Waisman, Y *et al.* 87
Wang, EE and Tang, NK 98, 99
Watson, RL *et al.* 116
Westley, CR *et al.* 82, 87
Williams, JW *et al.* 54
Williamson, HA *et al.* 107
work absenteeism 8, 15, 58
workload implications of ARIs 2–3, 9–10
World Health Organization, on EU
  antibiotic prescribing 127

zanamivir 71, 77
zinc
  as prophylactic measure 16, 19–20
  as treatment 17, 19–20
Zwar, N *et al.* 133